Mark Greener spent a decade in biomedical research before joining *MIMS*
M... for magazines w...
scientists. He's the author of 11 other bo...
in Adults (Sheldon Press, 2011). Mark lives with his wife,
two cats in a Cambridgeshire village.

Overcoming Common Problems Series

Selected titles

A full list of titles is available from Sheldon Press,
36 Causton Street, London SW1P 4ST and on our website at
www.sheldonpress.co.uk

101 Questions to Ask Your Doctor
Dr Tom Smith

Asperger Syndrome in Adults
Dr Ruth Searle

The Assertiveness Handbook
Mary Hartley

Assertiveness: Step by step
Dr Windy Dryden and Daniel Constantinou

Backache: What you need to know
Dr David Delvin

Birth Over 35
Sheila Kitzinger

Body Language: What you need to know
David Cohen

Bulimia, Binge-eating and their Treatment
Professor J. Hubert Lacey, Dr Bryony Bamford
and Amy Brown

The Cancer Survivor's Handbook
Dr Terry Priestman

The Chronic Pain Diet Book
Neville Shone

Cider Vinegar
Margaret Hills

Coeliac Disease: What you need to know
Alex Gazzola

Confidence Works
Gladeana McMahon

Coping Successfully with Pain
Neville Shone

Coping Successfully with Prostate Cancer
Dr Tom Smith

Coping Successfully with Psoriasis
Christine Craggs-Hinton

Coping Successfully with Ulcerative Colitis
Peter Cartwright

Coping Successfully with Varicose Veins
Christine Craggs-Hinton

Coping Successfully with Your Hiatus Hernia
Dr Tom Smith

Coping Successfully with Your Irritable Bowel
Rosemary Nicol

Coping When Your Child Has Cerebral Palsy
Jill Eckersley

Coping with Asthma in Adults
Mark Greener

**Coping with Birth Trauma and Postnatal
Depression**
Lucy Jolin

Coping with Bowel Cancer
Dr Tom Smith

Coping with Bronchitis and Emphysema
Dr Tom Smith

Coping with Candida
Shirley Trickett

Coping with Chemotherapy
Dr Terry Priestman

Coping with Chronic Fatigue
Trudie Chalder

Coping with Coeliac Disease
Karen Brody

Coping with Diverticulitis
Peter Cartwright

Coping with Drug Problems in the Family
Lucy Jolin

Coping with Dyspraxia
Jill Eckersley

Coping with Early-onset Dementia
Jill Eckersley

**Coping with Eating Disorders
and Body Image**
Christine Craggs-Hinton

Coping with Envy
Dr Windy Dryden

**Coping with Epilepsy in Children
and Young People**
Susan Elliot-Wright

Coping with Gout
Christine Craggs-Hinton

Coping with Hay Fever
Christine Craggs-Hinton

Coping with Headaches and Migraine
Alison Frith

Coping with Heartburn and Reflux
Dr Tom Smith

Coping with Kidney Disease
Dr Tom Smith

Overcoming Common Problems Series

Overcoming Common Problems Series

Overcoming Common Problems

The Heart Attack Survival Guide

MARK GREENER

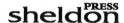

First published in Great Britain in 2012

Sheldon Press
36 Causton Street
London SW1P 4ST
www.sheldonpress.co.uk

British Library Cataloguing-in-Publication Data
A catalogue record for this book is available from the British Library

ISBN 978-1-84709-202-1
eBook ISBN 978-1-84709-203-8

Typeset by Fakenham Prepress Solutions, Fakenham, Norfolk NR21 8NN
Printed in Great Britain by Ashford Colour Press
Subsequently digitally printed in Great Britain

Produced on paper from sustainable forests

Contents

*To Rose, Yasmin, Rory and
Ophelia – with love*

Introduction

Every four minutes someone in the UK suffers a heart attack, according to the British Heart Foundation (BHF). So, each year, the National Health Service (NHS) manages around 124,000 heart attacks – most of which strike without warning. In 60 to 70 per cent of cases, the first sign of coronary heart disease (CHD) – the condition underlying most heart attacks – is sudden death or a myocardial infarction (MI), the medical term for a heart attack, as Gutterman noted in *Circulation Journal*.

Heart attacks kill, the BHF estimates, about 88,000 people a year – around one person every six minutes. In fact, CHD is the UK's leading cause of death, killing more people than lung, colorectal, breast and prostate cancer combined. (CHD includes angina and heart attacks, but not stroke or heart failure.) Worryingly, many people who suffer a heart attack die despite receiving advanced medical care. Between 11 and 12 per cent of men and 15 to 19 per cent of women die during the 30 days after they're admitted to hospital with a heart attack. Many other heart attack victims die before they even reach hospital.

Despite these sobering statistics, a heart attack isn't a death sentence. Improved treatments and greater awareness of risk factors among the public and health-care professionals have driven down deaths from heart disease over recent decades. Today, around 1 million men and almost 500,000 women are still alive after suffering heart attacks, the BHF estimates.

Yet, as thousands of funerals each year underscore, there's no room for complacency. Millions of people across the UK are at risk of suffering their first heart attack. And if you survive one heart attack, you may well face another. An MI is a symptom of CHD – and not the disease itself. So, a fifth of people who survive a heart attack suffer another MI in the next seven years, according to Haffner and colleagues. If you're one of the 2.8 million people with diagnosed diabetes in the UK (or one of the 850,000 who are unaware they have diabetes), your risk of having another heart attack after your first MI rises to almost 50 per cent – the chance of successfully calling heads when you flip a coin.

Everyone's at risk

Often CHD seems to be a disease of civilization. After all, we're more likely than our distant ancestors to stuff our faces with energy-dense, high-fat processed food, while puffing on cigarettes and rarely moving our overweight bodies from the sofa. Diet, obesity, smoking and inactivity are important modifiable risk factors for heart attacks. But atherosclerosis – the fatty deposits clogging up our blood vessels that cause most angina attacks and MIs – has lurked in our circulation for millennia.

In 1852, Johann Nepomuk Czermak, an Austrian–German scientist, found atherosclerosis in two ancient Egyptian mummies: a teenage boy and an elderly woman. More recently, Allam and colleagues found definite atherosclerosis in 12 of 44 ancient Egyptian mummies. Another eight mummies showed changes that probably indicated atherosclerosis. Two showed atherosclerosis in the blood vessels supplying the heart (the pattern responsible for heart attacks), including a princess who lived around 1580 to 1550 BC.

Indeed, atherosclerosis is present from the cradle to the grave. Foetuses may show fatty streaks smeared along the inside of their blood vessels. Doctors found atherosclerosis when they autopsied young, relatively fit men tragically killed during the Korean War. However, CHD typically takes decades to 'mature' and symptoms usually emerge in middle age and beyond. So, as this book shows, there's plenty of time to tackle heart disease – even if you've already developed angina, suffered a heart attack or are in your autumn years.

Breaking your heart

While almost anyone could suffer a heart attack, certain people are especially vulnerable. For example, cardiovascular disease kills just over half of people with type 2 diabetes. Stress, depression and other 'psychosocial' factors contribute to around a third of heart attacks. And everyone's exposed to traffic pollution, the most common heart attack trigger.

These risk factors 'cluster'. Hypertension (dangerously raised blood pressure), an important and common risk factor for MI, is between five and six times more common in obese people than in those of healthy weight. Around 40–60 per cent of people with type 2 diabetes have hypertension. But raised blood pressure increases MI risk whether you're chubby or lean and whether or not you have diabetes.

The more risk factors you have, the greater your chances of suffering a heart attack. According to INTERHEART – a major, worldwide investigation into MI risk factors – people with diabetes who smoke and have hypertension are 13 times more likely to suffer a heart attack than those without any of the three risk factors. Add a harmful profile of fat in your blood and obesity to these three risk factors and you're almost 69 times more likely to have a heart attack. People unfortunate enough to suffer psychosocial problems (such as severe stress at home or work, or depression) in addition to the five other risk factors are a massive 334 times more likely to suffer a heart attack than those without any of these risk factors.

This *Heart Attack Survival Guide* shows how you can reduce your blood pressure and cholesterol levels, quit smoking, lose weight and tackle stress – although you may need a helping hand from your doctor. The changes suggested in this book will dramatically improve your heart's health, help prevent your first MI and boost your chance of living a full life even if you've already suffered a heart attack or unstable angina – which is a dangerous 'first cousin' to MI. Remember that heart attacks are symptoms of an underlying disease. So, surviving long term means tackling the message – atherosclerosis – and not just the messenger (angina or MI).

Unfortunately, you can't do much about two other influential risk factors: age and sex. In England, around one man in every 167 and one woman in every 1,000 aged 35–44 years have experienced an MI, the BHF reports. The proportion rises to about one in six men and one in 11 women aged at least 75 years. Nevertheless, modifiable and unmodifiable factors interact to determine your overall risk. So tackling hypertension, stress, smoking and so on can reduce your chance of suffering a heart attack, whether you're young or old, male or female.

Heart disease risk and where you live

Heart attacks are 20–35 per cent more common in Scotland than south of the border. Deaths from CHD are highest in Scotland and the north of England and lowest in the south of England. The BHF notes that the number of premature deaths from CHD is 63 per cent higher in Scotland than in the south-west of England among men and 100 per cent higher among women. In Northern Ireland, deaths from CHD are around 20 per cent higher than in England among men and about 25 per cent higher among women. Heart disease deaths in Wales are around 15 per cent higher than in England for both sexes. Differences in several factors, including stress, diet, exercise and smoking, contribute to this variation.

Improve your chances

Wherever you live, whatever your age and whatever your risk factor profile, the *Heart Attack Survival Guide* helps you reduce your chances of suffering a heart attack. You'll need to change your lifestyle and, in many cases, take medicines as well. For example, INTERHEART found that not smoking reduces the risk of suffering your first heart attack by 65 per cent. Together, not smoking, eating fruit and vegetables daily, regular exercise and regular alcohol consumption cut MI risk by 81 per cent. (As we'll see, alcohol is a doubled-edged sword. It doesn't take many drinks before you risk damaging your health.) Drugs – despite their effectiveness – can't substitute for changing your lifestyle. But they're a life-saving safety net.

Changing your lifestyle is a long-term project. But you can take steps that immediately improve your prospects. Essentially, you need to prepare for the worst and make sure that your family and colleagues understand that calling 999 as soon as possible after you start suffering symptoms that might herald a heart attack could save your life. Indeed, rapid treatment is the most important step you can take to improve your chances of survival. According to NHS Choices, about 30 per cent of people who have a heart attack die before they reach hospital.

We'll see how a drug in almost every home's medicine box – aspirin – could save your life. We'll look at what happens once you reach A&E, including the drugs and operations to reopen blocked blood vessels that help you survive. We'll help heart attack survivors get back to a normal life as soon as possible after discharge from hospital. We'll look at some conditions that hinder a full recovery, how to tackle the heinous problem of depression and how to get back to work. And we'll look at how your partner can help you recover after an MI.

A heart attack isn't a death sentence. The *Heart Attack Survival Guide* shows that you can dramatically cut your chance of suffering an MI, often recover fully, and by tackling the underlying disease markedly reduce the risk that you'll have another heart attack. An MI doesn't need to break your heart.

A word to the wise

This book does not replace advice from cardiologists, GPs or nurses, who'll offer suggestions and support that are tailored to your circumstances. If you experience symptoms – such as a change in your pattern of angina – you should always consult your doctor as soon as possible.

The book includes numerous references from medical and scientific studies. But it's been impossible to cite them all. As you can imagine, researchers publish thousands of papers every year on heart disease. (Apologies to any researchers whose work I've missed.) However, throughout the book I've highlighted certain papers to illustrate key points and themes. If you want to know more about a particular study, I've given the reference in the back of the book. Some may seem rather erudite if you don't have a medical or biological background. But don't be put off. You can find a summary by entering the details here: <www.ncbi.nlm.nih.gov/pubmed>. In some cases, the full paper is available free on-line. Larger libraries may also stock or allow you to access on-line some of the better-known medical journals.

1

The heart of the matter

Unless our hearts pound 'fit to burst' as we try to keep up with the kids in the park, unless we suffer the crippling pain of angina, unless we end up in A&E after an MI, few of us think about the organ that beats in our chest hour after hour, day after day, year after year. Yet the heart is remarkable. At rest, a healthy heart typically pumps 60 to 80 times a minute, 86,000 to 115,000 times a day or around 3 billion times in 80 years, rarely missing a beat, without us thinking about it. So, to understand why heart attacks strike, why they're potentially so deadly and how to survive, we need to start by looking at a healthy heart and blood vessels – the cardiovascular system.

Your remarkable pump

On average, a healthy heart – which is about the size of your fist and weighs around 0.3 kilograms (10 ounces) – pumps 12 pints of blood along 60,000 miles of blood vessels. Incredibly, if you laid your blood vessels end-to-end they'd go around the equator almost two and a half times. Even at rest, a healthy heart pumps approximately 11,000 litres (2,500 gallons) of blood a day – shifting an Olympic swimming pool's worth of blood in about nine months. These blood vessels form two circulatory systems that begin and end at the heart (Figure 1.1):

- The pulmonary circulation connects your heart to your lungs.
- The systemic circulation connects your heart to all other parts of your body.

The heart is usually on the left side of the chest. Occasionally, the heart develops on the right side of the body (dextrocardia), which is often linked to defects in the cardiovascular system and other organs. However, around one in 7,000 people show 'situs inversus', where all their organs develop on the 'wrong' side of their body.

1

Apart from a slightly increased risk of heart defects, most people with *full* situs inversus live a normal life.

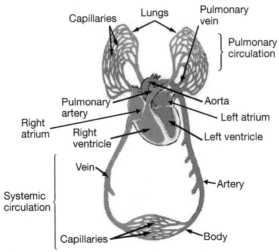

Figure 1.1 The circulatory system

The heart's four chambers – two atria and two ventricles (Figure 1.2) – beat in sequence, pushing blood around the circulation. Systole refers to the contraction of the heart's chambers. Diastole is the relaxation between beats, when the chambers fill with blood. That's why doctors and nurses record systolic and diastolic blood pressure (see page 29).

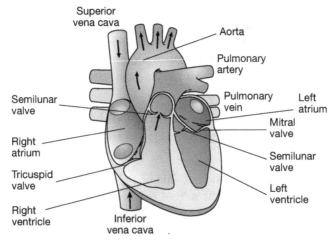

Figure 1.2 The structure of the heart

Atria and ventricles

The atria collect blood from the circulation. When they contract, the atria push blood into the ventricles. The two atria are smaller than the larger, stronger ventricles, with thinner, less muscular walls. Nevertheless, the atria help the ventricles work effectively. Some diseases – such as atrial fibrillation, when the atria beat up to 400 times per minute – mean that the heart doesn't pump blood properly. (As we'll see in Chapter 6, atrial fibrillation is common following heart attacks and dramatically cuts your chance of surviving.) Indeed, atrial fibrillation can reduce the amount of blood pumped by the heart by 15–20 per cent, Mulder and van der Wall remark.

The ventricles push blood around thousands of miles of blood vessels. The right atrium and right ventricle pump blood to the lungs. The left atrium and left ventricle pump blood around the systemic circulation. So, the left ventricle is more muscular than the right ventricle. The septum divides the left and right sides of the heart. Because it's much larger, around 70 per cent of heart attacks occur in the left ventricle.

The three layers of your heart wall

The walls of the heart contain three layers:

- The endocardium covers the inside of the heart, including the valves, and forms a continuous smooth layer with the inner lining of the blood vessels.
- The myocardium consists of thick bundles of cardiac muscle. Heart muscle occurs nowhere else in your body.
- The epicardium is the thin outer layer covering the outside of the heart.

Controlling the flow

Heart valves ensure that blood flows in the correct direction (see Figure 1.2):

- Tricuspid valves control the flow between the right atrium and right ventricle.
- Bicuspid (mitral) valves control the flow between the left atrium and left ventricle.

- Semilunar valves, which remind anatomists of a 'half moon', prevent blood that has been pumped into the arteries from flowing back into the ventricles.

Early in diastole, the pressure exerted by the blood in the atria opens the bicuspid valve and the tricuspid valve (together called the atrioventricular valves). Blood drains into the ventricles. As the volume of blood in the ventricles increases, squeezing more in becomes harder and harder. After about three-quarters of the blood has drained into the ventricles, the atrium contracts. This forces the remainder of the blood into the ventricles.

As the heart contracts, rising pressure in the ventricles closes the bicuspid and tricuspid valves. This prevents the pressure from forcing blood into the atria. As the pressure inside the ventricles increases further, the semilunar valves (sometimes called the pulmonary valve and the aortic valve) open. Blood flows into two large blood vessels: the pulmonary artery and the aorta. The semilunar valves close at the beginning of diastole, which prevents blood from flowing back into the ventricles.

Controlling the beat

Lurid stories of still-beating hearts cut from Aztec priests' sacrificial victims are mainstays of children's history programmes and popular documentaries on Mesoamerican cultures. It's more than a

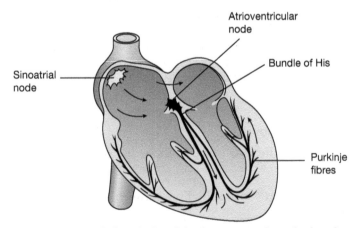

Figure 1.3 A wave of electrical activity keeps your heart's chambers beating in sequence

gory fairy story. Unlike every other muscle, your heart doesn't need stimulation from nerves to contract. A natural pacemaker generates the rhythm. The nervous system (along with some hormones) 'fine tunes' the rhythm to meet your body's needs.

This pacemaker – the sinus or sinoatrial node – lies in the wall of the right atrium. The sinoatrial node generates a pulse of electricity that spreads through the muscle to ensure that the heart contracts in sequence (Figure 1.3). Doctors measure this wave of electrical activity using an electrocardiogram (ECG).

The sinoatrial node starts each heartbeat and sets the pace. The impulse spreads from the sinoatrial node across both atria, which contract simultaneously. The impulse then reaches another pacemaker, called the atrioventricular node, which nestles in the wall separating the right and left atria. The atrioventricular node slows the impulse, allowing the atria sufficient time to finish pushing their loads of blood into the ventricles.

The electrical wave travels from the atrioventricular node along a collection of nerves called the bundle of His. (Wilhelm His, a Swiss doctor, discovered the eponymous structure in 1893.) The bundle of His (sometimes called the atrioventricular bundle) runs down the septum before splitting into right and left branches. The branches further divide into thousands of nerves. These nerves end in specialized muscle cells, called Purkinje fibres, found throughout the ventricles. The Purkinje fibres trigger the ventricles' contraction.

The circulatory system

Blood from the body, rich in carbon dioxide, enters the right atrium through two large veins: the superior vena cava and the inferior vena cava (see Figure 1.2). The right atrium pumps blood into the right ventricle. When the heart contracts, blood flows from the right ventricle into the pulmonary artery (also called the pulmonary trunk). This artery divides into the right pulmonary artery and the left pulmonary artery, each supplying one of the two lungs.

The difference between arteries, veins and capillaries

Arteries carry blood away *from* the heart and branch into medium-sized and then small arteries (arterioles). These 'arterioles' divide into capillaries: a network of microscopic vessels inside all your body's tissues from your skin to your deepest internal organs. Capillaries' thin walls allow oxygen and nutrients to move from the blood into the cells. Meanwhile, blood in the capillaries absorbs carbon dioxide and other waste products. (In the lung, oxygen moves *into* the capillaries, while carbon dioxide moves out.) Capillaries merge, forming venules and, in turn, veins that return blood *to* the heart. Most arteries carry oxygen-rich blood. Most veins carry oxygen-depleted blood. However, pulmonary arteries carry oxygen-poor blood from your heart to your lungs. Pulmonary veins return oxygen-rich blood to your heart.

In the lungs, carbon dioxide moves from the blood into the alveoli. We expel toxic carbon dioxide when we breathe out. Meanwhile, oxygen in the air we've breathed in moves from the alveoli and attaches to an iron-rich protein (haemoglobin) in red blood cells (erythrocytes). Oxygen-rich blood travels from the lung through four pulmonary veins to the left atrium.

The muscular left ventricle pumps blood into the ascending aorta (see Figure 1.2). From here, the blood takes one of four routes:

- Coronary arteries – although the atria and ventricles are full of blood, the heart needs a network of vessels to supply the heart (cardiac) muscle with oxygen and nutrients. Angina's crippling chest pain occurs when the heart's demand for oxygen outstrips supply from the coronary arteries. Most heart attacks occur after a blockage in the coronary circulation stops this essential blood flow. So, the cardiac muscle supplied by the vessel dies.
- Carotid arteries carry blood along the neck to the brain and into the cerebral circulation. Ischaemic strokes (page 31) arise from blockages in the cerebral circulation.
- The thoracic aorta supplies organs in the chest, the head, the arms and hands.
- The abdominal aorta supplies organs between the chest and pelvis as well as the legs and feet.

Inside your lungs

After entering your mouth and nose, air flows along your trachea, which is about 10–16 cm long and around 2 cm wide. Horseshoe-shaped rings of cartilage – rather like the rings on a vacuum cleaner hose – protect the trachea from crushing. The trachea forks into two major bronchi, one supplying each lung. Each major bronchus divides another 10–25 times into bronchi and then bronchioles. The bronchioles end in between 300 million and 500 million alveoli, which look like cauliflower florets. The bronchial tree's shape packs a vast area into a relatively small volume. Overall, our lungs contain approximately 1,500 miles of airways. In an adult, the alveoli's surface area is about 70 square metres – roughly the same as a single tennis court. A network of around 620 miles of capillaries surrounds the alveoli.

Controlling heart rate

The cardiac pacemakers allow your heart to beat independently of nervous control. However, your nervous system helps 'fine tune' the rate and force of the heartbeat. Your brain and spinal cord make up your central nervous system (CNS). Biologists divide nerves outside the CNS – the peripheral nervous system – into two parts:

- The 'somatic' or 'voluntary' nervous system, which allows us to choose our actions. Your voluntary nervous system told your muscles to turn the pages of this book, for example.
- The 'autonomic' or 'involuntary' nervous system, which keeps essential bodily functions – such as breathing and heartbeat – going without conscious control, such as while we're asleep. It's easy to decide to pick up a pen, harder to slow your pounding heart before a presentation. However, yoga, meditation, biofeedback and several other techniques may allow you to exert some control over your autonomic nerves.

Biologists divide the autonomic nervous system into sympathetic and parasympathetic nerves. These have opposite actions. For example:

- Sympathetic nerves increase the rate and force of the heartbeat. Sympathetic nerves also open the coronary arteries to increase the supply of oxygen and nutrients to fuel the heart's increased activity.

- Parasympathetic nerves slow heart rate, reduce the force of contraction and narrow (constrict) the coronary arteries.

The balance between sympathetic and parasympathetic nervous activity largely determines heart rate. However, some hormones – such as adrenaline, released from the adrenal glands on top of your kidneys – further 'fine tune' the speed and force of contraction.

Without the influence of the autonomic nervous system and hormones, the sinoatrial node produces a resting heart rate of between 100 and 120 beats per minute (bpm). Usually, parasympathetic activity reduces resting heart rate to, typically, between 60 and 80 bpm. However, numerous factors influence heart rate. For example:

- When you face stress or danger, sympathetic activity increases. Apart from their effects on the heart, sympathetic nerves stimulate your adrenal glands to secrete adrenaline and other hormones that increase blood pressure and heart rate.
- Changes in respiratory rate (breaths each minute) can alter heart rate by 12 to 15 bpm. That's why taking deep breaths can help you feel calmer. As more oxygen reaches your blood your heart doesn't need to work as hard. Nerves tell your brain that the heart's rate and force has declined. The 'feedback' means that it's hard to feel mentally stressed when your body relaxes. And you feel mentally calmer.
- Physical fitness can influence heart rate. Occasionally, for example, an unfit, sedentary person will have a resting heart rate of over 100 bpm. In contrast, some endurance athletes have resting heart rates of just 30 bpm.

More than plumbing

Your circulatory system is your body's largest organ. Taken together, your blood vessels weigh about five times more than your heart. But blood vessels are more than simple pipes. They consist of three layers, which allow your vessels to respond to your body's demands:

- the tunica intima (literally 'inside coat', the smooth inner lining;

- the tunica media, the middle layer, which controls the vessel's diameter and maintains its flexibility; and
- the tunica adventitia (or tunica externa), which maintains the vessel's shape, limits distension and anchors the vessel to nearby organs.

Each heartbeat generates sufficient force to send a fountain of blood spurting several feet into the air. So, the tunica media in arteries is much thicker than in veins to withstand the force of blood pumped from the heart. Arteries also expand to accommodate the surge of blood. Your pulse is the pressure wave generated as blood travels along the arteries.

As the arteries divide into arterioles and then capillaries, blood pressure gradually weakens. By the time the capillaries join to form venules and veins, there's little pressure left to push blood back to the heart against gravity. So, the tunica intima of veins folds over, forming valves. These valves prevent blood from flowing back towards your ankles. Weak or damaged valves allow blood to flow backwards, causing varicose (enlarged, swollen) veins.

This chapter has briefly looked at a healthy cardiovascular system. Now we'll see what happens when you suffer a heart attack.

2

When a heart attack strikes

Around 500 years ago, Leonardo da Vinci noticed that a layer of 'waxy fat' covered elderly people's coronary vessels. Today, we know that fat starts collecting *inside* arteries from early childhood – perhaps even while we are in the womb. This accumulation – atherosclerosis – is the main cause of heart attacks.

'Sclerosis' means hardening, and *athere* is the Greek word for gruel or porridge, which gives you an idea of the consistency. I'll never forget the film at a medical conference where a cardiac surgeon ran his finger along the outside of an artery with severe atherosclerosis. Fat ran out of the end as if he was squeezing toothpaste from a tube.

The 'gruel' kills more people in the UK than any other condition. Cardiovascular diseases claim almost 191,000 lives a year, the BHF estimates – one in three deaths – in the UK. CHD accounts for almost half of deaths from cardiovascular disease. Strokes cause just under a quarter. Other less common conditions make up the remainder.

The grim reaper's changing face

In 1880, infections and parasites caused a third of deaths. Only one in 10 people died from circulatory diseases and cancer. By 1961, cardiovascular diseases accounted for more than half of all deaths. Indeed, by 1961, cardiovascular disease was the biggest killer at all ages from 35 years up. Since then, deaths from heart disease have declined. For example, between 1998 and 2008, deaths from CHD in people aged 55 to 64 years roughly halved.

From the cradle to the grave

Atherosclerosis starts as a 'smear' of fat along the inside of a blood vessel. Some foetuses show these fatty streaks. However, the number of fatty streaks increases dramatically from about 8 years of age. Most people have fatty streaks in their aorta and coronary arteries by their 20th birthday.

Plaques usually start developing at around 25 years of age and often take between 10 and 15 years to mature fully. So symptoms (such as angina or intermittent claudication – see below) tend to start to appear in middle age. As a plaque enlarges, the lumen (the size of the 'bore' down the middle of the vessel) narrows (Figure 2.1). This reduces the blood flow to the organ the vessel supplies. The reduced blood supply can cause a range of health problems depending on the site of the plaque, including chest pain (angina), kidney damage and even impotence (see Chapter 8).

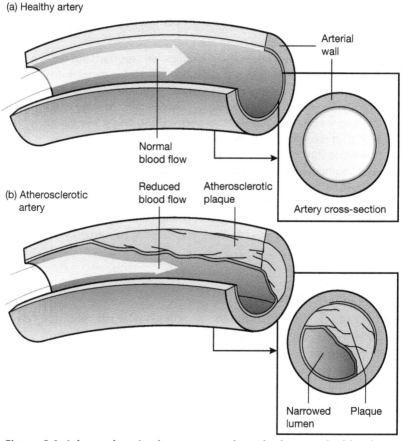

(a) Healthy artery

Arterial wall

Normal blood flow

Artery cross-section

(b) Atherosclerotic artery

Reduced blood flow

Atherosclerotic plaque

Narrowed lumen

Plaque

Figure 2.1 Atherosclerotic plaques can reduce the lumen of a blood vessel

Peripheral artery disease refers to atherosclerosis in vessels other than the coronary circulation. A plaque in the coronary circulation (known as coronary artery disease) reduces blood flow to the heart. Exercise and stress increase the heart's demand for oxygen. So, a plaque can trigger chest pain during exercise or when you're emotionally stressed (stable angina). The pain forces you to rest or calm down, which rebalances supply and demand.

Peripheral artery disease

In peripheral arterial disease, atherosclerotic plaques develop in arteries supplying your head, kidneys, stomach and other organs, and limbs. For example, the reduced blood supply to your legs – the most common site of peripheral atherosclerosis – can cause intermittent claudication (from the Latin for 'to limp').

People who have intermittent claudication report aching or cramping pain, with tightness or fatigue in their leg muscles or buttocks. Some people find that the pain arises only during strenuous activity. People with more severe peripheral arterial disease may develop intermittent claudication after walking only a few metres. The pain subsides after a few minutes' rest. Severe blockages to the blood flow can cause gangrene (tissue death), which may even end in amputation. One person in every three with coronary artery disease has peripheral arterial disease affecting the legs, which can emerge before chest symptoms. In other words, intermittent claudication may be a warning that you're especially likely to suffer a heart attack. So, tell your doctor if you have leg pain when you walk or climb stairs.

Clots and heart attacks

In 1844, Bertel Thorvaldsen, a famous Danish sculptor, died suddenly at the Copenhagen Royal Theatre. The autopsy on Thorvaldsen's body revealed several artrerosclerotic plaques in his coronary arteries. One plaque, the doctor memorably described, had 'quite clearly . . . ulcerated, pouring the atheromatous mass into the arterial lumen'.

As Thorvaldsen's doctor discovered, when an atherosclerotic plaque bursts or cracks, the contents spill into the vessel and trigger a blood clot. In the coronary circulation, the blood clot partially or totally blocks the vessel, starving your heart of blood and oxygen. A severe decline in supply damages and then kills the muscle supplied by the vessel. Doctors call the inadequate oxygen supply 'ischaemia'. So ischaemic symptoms or ischaemic heart disease arise from the lack of oxygen. Blood can also carry clots or plaque fragments from arteries elsewhere in the body, which can stick in the coronary circulation. However, these 'embolisms' are a less common cause of heart attacks than ruptured plaques.

Ischaemic symptoms – such as angina, intermittent claudication and even impotence – should act as a 'wake-up call' warning you to improve your cardiovascular health. However, when a coronary artery narrows, other nearby vessels may expand to keep the heart supplied with oxygen. This 'collateral circulation' is one reason why the large plaques responsible for stable angina rarely cause heart attacks. Most plaques that rupture and cause heart attacks block less than half the blood vessel and may not cause angina. Indeed, Gutterman notes, in 60 to 70 per cent of cases, sudden death or a heart attack is the first sign of coronary artery disease. Doctors call unexpected mortality from heart disease – such as cardiac arrest (see below) – 'sudden death'. Almost half of CHD deaths are sudden.

Introducing a heart attack's symptoms

Heart attack symptoms vary from person to person. Some people experience severe pain, a dull ache or 'heavy' feeling in their chest. Other people suffer only mild discomfort – similar to bad indigestion. The pain or discomfort may spread to the arms, neck, jaw, back or stomach. Some heart attack victims feel light-headed or dizzy, breathless or nauseous or may vomit. Chapter 4 looks at a heart attack's symptoms in detail. You MUST call 999 for an ambulance immediately – don't phone your GP or NHS Direct first – if you think you or anyone else is having a heart attack: rapid treatment is the most important step you can take to increase the chances of survival.

Cardiac arrest

A heart attack is *not* the same as cardiac arrest. During a cardiac arrest, the heart stops pumping blood. You'll lose consciousness almost immediately and won't breathe normally.

Several events can trigger cardiac arrest, including heart attacks, electrocution, choking, losing large amounts of blood, being very hot or cold, and ventricular fibrillation. Heart attacks can also cause ventricular fibrillation.

During ventricular fibrillation, the most common cause of cardiac arrest, the heart's electrical activity becomes chaotic. The ventricles stop pumping and 'quiver' (fibrillate). Defibrillators deliver an electric shock through the chest wall, which sometimes restores normal beats. Without cardiopulmonary resuscitation and defibrillation, most cardiac arrests kill. If you think someone is in cardiac arrest, call 999 immediately and give cardiopulmonary resuscitation.

Plaque development

Atherosclerosis is the leading cause of heart attacks. So it's worth looking at a plaque's development in more detail (Figure 2.2). Plaques begin as smears of fat that form around damage to the tunica intima, the blood vessel's normally smooth inner lining. For example, atherosclerosis can develop where blood flow is particularly turbulent, such as at branches in medium and large blood vessels. And, as we'll see in Chapter 3, numerous risk factors can damage the delicate tunica intima and sow the seeds of atherosclerosis, including:

- excessive levels of fat in the blood (dyslipidaemia);
- raised sugar levels in the blood (diabetes);

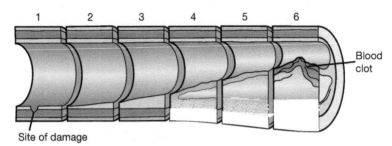

Blood clot

Site of damage
1 Damage to the inner lining of the blood vessel
2 Fatty streak forms at site of damage
3 Foam cells numbers increase, area is inflamed and small pools of fat appear
4 Large core of fat develops, and amounts of muscle and collagen increase
5 Fibrous cap covers a fat-rich core, while calcium deposits harden the plaque
6 Plaque ruptures triggering a blood clot

Figure 2.2 Development of an atherosclerotic plaque

- dangerously high blood pressure (hypertension);
- changes linked to age;
- nicotine and other toxins from smoking; and
- inflammation that spills over from diseases in other parts of the body.

Damage to the tunica intima allows fats and certain types of white blood cell to enter the vessel wall. Some of the white blood cells engorge with fat, forming foam cells. Meanwhile, chemicals released by white blood cells promote inflammation around the damaged area and increase the amount of muscle and collagen in the blood vessel wall. (Collagen, which accounts for about a quarter of the protein in your body, enhances tissues' strength and flexibility.) The chemicals also recruit even more white blood cells into the damaged area.

These changes help 'patch' the damaged vessel wall. But it's a short term 'fix'. As fat continues to pour from the blood into the plaque, muscle cells form a fibrous cap covering a core of foam cells, lipid and debris from dead cells. Capillaries grow into the developing plaque. But these vessels are fragile. So, blood leaks into, and further swells, the plaque. Calcium deposits gradually harden the plaque.

A silent killer

At first, coronary arteries enlarge to accommodate the plaque. But after the plaque occupies more than 40 per cent of the vessel wall, it begins to narrow the lumen and cuts blood flow. Once a plaque blocks at least 50–70 per cent of the lumen, blood flow falls sufficiently to produce angina in many people. Doctors describe a severe narrowing as stenosis.

However, in some people, even marked declines in blood flow don't cause symptoms. Overall, between 2 and 4 per cent of us show this 'silent ischaemia' from time-to-time, a figure that can reach 80–100 per cent among heart attack survivors. Gutterman notes that, following a heart attack, silent ischaemia increases by almost three times the risk of suffering a further major cardiac event – such as death, another MI or the need for bypass surgery – over the next year.

Even heart attacks can be 'silent'. In other words, a person may show the changes in ECG, blood tests and so on (see Chapter 4) that are characteristic of a heart attack but not the symptoms. In other people, the discomfort is so mild that they dismiss the sensation as, for instance, indigestion. In such cases, the patient receives the bad news that he or she has suffered a heart attack after undergoing a test for another problem or during a 'routine' check up.

Darren's story

Darren – a 48-year-old banker – enjoyed a curry, usually washed down with a few beers after work on a Friday. He regarded a bout of indigestion on Saturday morning as the wages of his indulgence. But one morning, the antacids didn't work. His wife's father died from a heart attack. Darren said he'd be all right in a while. But his wife insisted on calling for an ambulance. The doctor in A&E told them Darren had suffered a heart attack.

Plaque rupture

Some plaques remain unchanged for years. In other cases, inflammation weakens the fibrous cap. So, the plaque becomes unstable, especially where the cap meets the vessel wall. Once the plaque has weakened sufficiently, trigger factors, such as exercise, increased blood pressure or changes in the vessel diameter, can rupture the plaque. Plaque rupture causes approximately 70 per cent of heart attacks and cases of unstable angina, a related disease discussed below. Most other heart attacks follow the cap's slow erosion, Corrales-Medina and colleagues remark.

Most plaques responsible for heart attacks block less than half of the blood vessel's diameter. However, these smaller plaques contain relatively more fat in their core and the fibrous cap is thinner than in large stable plaques. So, smaller plaques are more likely to burst and trigger a clot that, if it completely blocks the coronary vessels, results in a heart attack. A clot that does not entirely block the vessel can cause unstable angina.

During an MI, oxygen starvation damages and then kills heart muscle. Stable angina develops when the heart's demand for oxygen outstrips supply – such as during exercise or intense emotion. However, in stable angina no clot blocks the vessel, resting restores the balance and the heart muscle isn't damaged. Unstable angina occurs when a clot partially blocks the vessel and resting doesn't restore the balance, but the heart isn't damaged.

Unstable angina produces similar symptoms to stable angina. However, unstable angina typically emerges at rest, and is more severe and prolonged – usually lasting longer than 20 minutes – than stable angina. Such symptoms are important warning signs. About 30 per cent of people have a heart attack within three months of suffering unstable angina. Moreover, between 5 and 8 per cent of people die within six months of experiencing unstable angina. This compares to a death rate of 12 to 15 per cent following a heart attack, Rogowski and co-authors say. Indeed, the risk of death and a further MI over the longer term may be higher following unstable angina than after many heart attacks.

If you suffer symptoms that could be unstable angina (whether or not you've previously suffered a heart attack) you should go to A&E. You should tell your doctor immediately (or go to A&E) if your pattern of angina changes, such as from symptoms after exercise to symptoms while watching the television. Nevertheless, even experienced doctors using the latest diagnostic techniques (see Chapter 4) sometimes can't distinguish a heart attack from unstable angina. So, your doctor may tell you that you have an 'acute coronary syndrome', a term that encompasses heart attacks and unstable angina.

Limiting the damage

In around two-thirds of heart attacks and episodes of unstable angina, the body removes the obstruction within 24 hours. Meanwhile, the body repairs the damaged plaque and nearby vessels (the collateral circulation) may expand. This collateral circulation helps heart muscle recover. And doctors can open blocked arteries using drugs and surgery (see Chapter 5). But time is of the essence. A blockage of coronary arteries that lasts for more than 20 minutes starts irreversibly damaging the heart.

The larger the area supplied by the blocked vessel, the more severe the damage. At first, the edge of the area of heart muscle (which receives the least blood) supplied by the artery dies. If the blockage persists, the area of cell death (technically called necrosis) enlarges, so that eventually even areas previously well supplied with blood die. Eventually, necrosis extends through the heart's three layers (a transmural MI) and spreads sideways. If the blockage lasts between six and eight hours, most of the muscle supplied by the vessel has died. But rapidly restoring blood flow – for example using drugs or surgery to unblock the artery – can limit the damage. That's why it's so important to ensure you're treated quickly.

A few days after the heart attack, scar tissue begins to replace the damaged muscle. In many cases, the heart recovers fully after two or three months, the BHF comments. However, scar tissue does not contract as well as healthy muscle, which in some people, leads to breathlessness, tiredness and swollen ankles – the hallmarks of heart failure (see page 74). The scar may also cause tell-tale changes on ECGs.

Although the body may repair the damage and although doctors can restore the blood supply, many plaques remain unstable. Furthermore, few heart attack survivors have a single plaque. So, people who have had a heart attack are at high risk of suffering another MI. That means to survive long term you need to tackle the underlying disease.

Heart attack triggers

Heart attack triggers are distinct from the risk factors that we'll consider in Chapter 3. Triggers increase the risk of a heart attack within the next few hours. Risk factors increase the likelihood of suffering a heart attack by acting over several years. For example, Tofler and colleagues found that in about one in five cases, heart attacks occurred during physical activity. However, over the long term, exercise is one of the best ways to prevent a heart attack.

Nawrot and co-workers analysed 36 studies assessing the risk of suffering a heart attack between two hours and a day after encountering a variety of triggers. (They made an exception for respiratory infections, when the window was one to 10 days before the heart attack.) Cocaine increased heart attack risk 24 times (Table 2.1). Cocaine is a very powerful stimulant that dramatically increases the force and speed of the heartbeat. Other triggers included a heavy meal (a seven-fold increase), exercise (a four-fold increase) and sex (a three-fold increase). A heavy meal, for example, increases heart rate and blood pressure, both of which can rupture plaques. Eating also triggers a rise in insulin (the hormone that tells your cells to take up glucose from the blood). The more you eat, the

Table 2.1 Increased risk of heart attack associated with certain triggers

Trigger	Odds ratio
Cocaine use	23.7
Heavy meal	7.0
Marijuana use	4.8
Negative emotions	4.5
Physical exercise	4.3
Positive emotions	3.5
Anger	3.1
Alcohol	3.1
Sexual activity	3.1
Traffic exposure	2.9
Respiratory infection	2.7
Coffee	1.5
Air pollution	1.02–1.05

Odds ratios measure how more likely someone exposed to the trigger is to suffer a heart attack compared to someone who is not exposed. An odds ratio of 3 means that they are three times more likely to suffer a heart attack.

Source: Nawrot and co-workers.

more insulin you produce. However, insulin hinders the coronary arteries' ability to dilate to increase blood flow in response to the faster heart rate.

Table 2.1 shows the most important risk factors for individuals. But that's not the same as the most important trigger for the population *as a whole*. For example, cocaine carries the greatest risk. However, only one person in every 2,500 uses cocaine, Nawrot and colleagues comment. On the other hand, air pollution slightly increases the risk – by 2–5 per cent. But everyone is exposed. Taking into account the risk for the individual *and* the number of people exposed, air pollution is the most common trigger, followed by physical exertion, coffee and alcohol.

Watching for triggers can help you avoid situations that could precipitate a heart attack. It's probably best to avoid a heavy meal washed down with copious amounts of alcohol and strong coffee, for example. When you go on holiday (see Chapter 8), avoid heavily polluted cities and hotels perched on the top of steep hills. And get your flu jab each year (see Chapter 7). Respiratory infections occur shortly before up to a third of episodes of acute coronary syndrome, Corrales-Medina and co-authors note. The risk is almost five-fold higher in the first 72 hours and may remain raised for up to three months.

A daily rhythm

The risk of suffering a heart attack peaks in the morning, with a smaller peak in late evening. Sudden death, angina and silent ischaemia show similar patterns:

- Hjalmarson and colleagues found that 28 per cent of heart attacks occurred between 6:01 a.m. and noon, a rate 16 per cent higher than the average at other times. Another 25 per cent of heart attacks occurred between 6:01 p.m. and midnight.
- Tofler and co-authors found that the number of heart attacks was 34 per cent higher between 6.00 a.m. and noon than at other times of the day.
- Cohen and co-workers analysed several studies and found that the risk of suffering a heart attack was 40 per cent higher between 6.00 a.m. and noon.

Several factors contribute to this daily (diurnal or circadian) rhythm. Obviously, you're physically and mentally more active when you wake than while you're asleep. So, heart rate and blood pressure rise. Patel and colleagues comment that blood pressure dips by 10–20 per cent during the night and then increases just before you wake up. Blood's propensity to clot also peaks between 6.00 a.m. and 9.00 p.m.

The early morning changes prepare our body for the hazards we could encounter during the day. Faster clotting protects us from bleeding excessively if we're injured, for example. As Hjalmarson and colleagues note, the reasons for an evening peak are less obvious, but they may include altered rhythms due to late working hours. And some of us may naturally be 'owls' rather than 'larks'. While there's little you can do about these biological rhythms, some lifestyle changes and long-acting drugs protect against these peaks.

Anaemia and heart attacks

Depending on the characteristics of the people studied and the definitions used, between 6 and 43 per cent of those who have had a heart attack have anaemia, Anker and colleagues remark. People with anaemia have too little haemoglobin, the iron-containing protein in red blood cells (erythrocytes) that carries oxygen. For instance, some anaemic people produce too few red blood cells. Each red blood cell lives for 100 to 120 days. The body destroys old, inefficient red blood cells. However, some people destroy too many healthy red blood cells, resulting in anaemia. Other causes include deficiencies in vitamin B_{12}, iron or folic acid (which result in abnormal blood cell production), long-lasting inflammation and certain cancers.

The symptoms of anaemia arise from a mismatch between the demand for oxygen by tissues and the supply. As a result, anaemic people may feel fatigued and weak or suffer headache and palpitations. If they breathe normally, the body 'senses' that oxygen levels are too low. So, they feel breathless – a trigger to inhale more oxygen – and exercise becomes more difficult. Low haemoglobin levels further undermine oxygen supply, which exacerbates any damage to the heart. Anaemia can also cause severe chest pain, again because the heart receives insufficient oxygen. So, the heart works harder and the left ventricle thickens (left ventricular hypertrophy – see page 75).

Indeed, anaemia increases the risk of death among people with heart failure and after a heart attack. In a year-long study, Anker and colleagues found that heart attack survivors who developed heart failure and showed anaemia were 35 per cent more likely to die during the trial than those with normal haemoglobin levels. People with anaemia were 31 per cent more likely to be hospitalized for heart failure and 55 per cent more likely to die after heart failure progressed. On the other hand, increasing haemoglobin reduced deaths by 27 per cent even in people who had anaemia at the start of the study.

So, if you've suffered a heart attack or symptoms, such as intermittent claudication or angina, it is probably worth asking your doctor to measure your haemoglobin level. You could also consider taking a multivitamin or – even better – eating foods rich in vitamin

B_{12}, iron or folic acid (see Chapter 7). Ask your GP or a dietician or the look at the British Dietetic Association website if you're unsure.

What's my chance of surviving a heart attack?

Early treatment dramatically boosts your chance of surviving a heart attack. According to NHS Choices, treatment should ideally begin within 90 minutes of symptoms emerging. Nevertheless, just over half of people who have a heart attack die within 28 days. Of these, 75 per cent die in the first 24 hours. Thirty per cent of the deaths occur even before the person reaches hospital. On the other hand, if you survive for 28 days after your heart attack, you'll probably live for many more years, especially if you and your doctor work together to tackle your risk factors, the subject of the next chapter.

3

Risk factors for heart attacks

Surf the internet, flick through a medical textbook or read magazines and newspapers, and it's easy to feel that almost anything increases your chance of suffering a heart attack. Indeed, depending on who does the counting, doctors have identified between 200 and 300 risk factors for heart disease. So, where do you start – especially as some risk factors seem bizarre?

For example, men with mild baldness on the top of their heads ('the vertex pattern') were 23 per cent more likely to develop CHD during the next 11 years than those with fuller heads of hair, according to Lotufo and colleagues. Moderate and severe vertex baldness increased the risk by 32 per cent and 36 per cent, respectively. Another study found that people with creased ear lobes are more likely to develop CHD. Christoffersen and colleagues found that adults with flat yellow 'spots' on their upper or lower eyelids (xanthelasmata) were 69 per cent more likely to develop severe atherosclerosis over an average of 22 years, 48 per cent more likely to suffer a heart attack, 39 per cent more likely to suffer ischaemic heart disease and 14 per cent more likely to die.

Age, sex and heart attacks

Men are more likely to die from CHD, stroke and other cardiovascular diseases than women. However, women tend to live longer. So, the total number of deaths from these diseases is similar. The risk of suffering a heart attack rises rapidly with age in both men and women. In England, one in 167 men and one in 1,000 women aged 35–44 years have experienced a heart attack, the BHF report. Among men, the proportion who have suffered a heart attack increases to one in 50 between 45 and 54 years of age and to around one in six of those 75 years of age and over. In women, the proportion increases to one in 62 between 55 and 64 years of age and about one in 11 of those 75 years of age and over.

But dig a little deeper and these seemingly strange risk factors start making sense. High levels of androgens – male sex hormones, such as testosterone – seem to increase the risk of baldness. And androgens boost the likelihood of suffering CHD. Age-related changes in proteins seem to cause the ear lobe crease, suggesting the person is ageing rapidly. Similar biological mechanisms probably cause both xanthelasmata and atherosclerotic plaques.

You can't do much about some heart attack risk factors – such as your age, your pattern of baldness and your sex. But nine easily measured and potentially modifiable risk factors account for about nine in every 10 first heart attacks. As the INTERHEART study illustrates, lifestyle changes targeting these nine risk factors dramatically cut your chances of suffering your first or another heart attack. For example, not smoking and avoiding dangerous levels of fats in the blood would prevent around two-thirds of first heart attacks. However, remember that a heart attack is a symptom caused by cardiovascular disease. So, increasing your chances of surviving long term means tackling the heart attack risk factors.

The INTERHEART study: the risk factors that matter

These nine factors emerged from the landmark INTERHEART study, which compared 15,152 people from 52 countries who'd suffered their first heart attack with 14,820 people who'd never experienced an MI. The nine factors accounted for 90 per cent of the risk of the first heart attack among men and 94 per cent among women. The factors had, broadly, the same impact in men and women, the same impact across different geographic regions and the same impact among different ethnic groups.

INTERHEART looked at the risk of the first heart attack. But the same principles apply to further heart attacks after your first MI – as we'll see. Indeed, because you're at higher risk, the benefits of addressing the risk factors are likely to be even greater.

Smoking almost trebled the chances of suffering a MI. Smoking just one to five cigarettes a day increased the risk by 38 per cent compared to lifelong non-smokers. The risk roughly doubled in those smoking six to 10 cigarettes a day, increased almost four-fold between 16 and 20 a day, and rose to just over nine-fold in people smoking at least 41 cigarettes a day.

INTERHEART also found that diabetes and hypertension each roughly doubled the risk of the first heart attack. High levels of harmful fats in the blood increased MI risk up to three-fold (Table 3.1). Abdominal obesity ('a bulging waistline') increased the risk by between 12 and 62 per cent. Finally, psychosocial factors (such as stress and depression) roughly trebled the risk.

On the other hand, eating fruits and vegetables daily (30 per cent reduction), regular exercise (14 per cent reduction) and regular alcohol consumption (9 per cent reduction) protected against the first heart attack. Chapter 7 looks at how you can make these heart healthy factors part of your everyday life.

To look at the factors from another angle, researchers estimated the 'population attributable risk' (PAR). The PAR refers to the proportion of MIs in the population caused by the risk factor. The PAR for current and former smoking was about 36 per cent. In other words, eliminating smoking would prevent more than a third of first MIs. The PAR for high levels of harmful fats in the blood was around 49 per cent. So eliminating abnormal fat levels would halve the number of first heart attacks. Hypertension (18 per cent) and abdominal obesity (20 per cent) accounted for almost a fifth of MIs, and diabetes for one in ten first heart attacks (10 per cent).

Unfortunately, many heart attack risk factors 'cluster'. So, if you eat a high-fat diet, you're more likely to be overweight or obese. If you're overweight or obese you're more likely to develop diabetes, hypertension or both. Not surprisingly, the more risk factors you have the greater your chance of suffering a heart attack:

- People with diabetes who smoke and have hypertension are 13 times more likely to suffer a heart attack than those without any of the nine risk factors.
- Those with five risk factors (harmful fat levels, obesity, smoking, diabetes and hypertension) are almost 69 times more likely to have a heart attack.
- If you're unfortunate enough to suffer psychosocial factors in addition to these other five risk factors you are about 334 times more likely to suffer a heart attack than those without any of the nine risk factors.

Table 3.1 Factors linked to the risk of suffering the first heart attack in the INTERHEART study

Risk factors	Increase in risk of MI
Hypertension alone	1.9 times
Diabetes alone	2.4 times
Smoking alone	2.9 times
Abnormal lipid profile (ApoB/A1 ratio) *	3.3 times
Hypertension, diabetes, smoking	13.0 times
Hypertension, diabetes, smoking, adverse lipids	42.3 times
Hypertension, diabetes, smoking, adverse lipids, obesity	68.5 times
Hypertension, diabetes, smoking, adverse lipids, psychosocial factors	182.9 times
Hypertension, diabetes, smoking, adverse lipids, psychosocial factors, obesity	333.7 times

* See page 34 for an explanation.

Stress and psychological factors

We've seen that emotions can trigger angina and heart attacks. INTERHEART assessed the link between stress – which the researchers defined as feeling irritable, filled with anxiety or having difficulty sleeping because of problems – and heart attacks. The researchers looked at stress over the year before the study and separated, as far as possible:

- stress at work;
- stress at home;
- stress caused by financial problems; and
- major stressful life events (such as divorce, business failure, unemployment or death of a spouse).

The analysis allowed for the impact of other risk factors, such as age, sex and smoking. (You may smoke more if you're stressed out, for example.) They found that:

- People who experienced several periods of work-related stress were 38 per cent more likely to suffer a heart attack.
- Experiencing several periods of stress at home increased the risk of an MI by 52 per cent.

- Heart attack risk roughly doubled among those who endured permanent stress at work or home.
- Severe financial stress increased the likelihood of suffering a first MI by 33 per cent.
- Stressful life events increased first MI risk by 48 per cent.

Feeling depressed for at least last two weeks in the year before the study increased MI risk by 55 per cent. As we'll see in Chapter 6, depression can also dramatically reduce your chances of surviving a heart attack.

On the other hand, feeling that you control your life protects against heart attacks and helps you cope with crises in general. Psychologists describe the extent to which you feel you control your life as your 'locus of control'. If you have a strong external locus of control, you see yourself as having little influence over your life. You feel that events control you, you don't control events. A strong internal locus of control means you tend to see yourself as in charge of your life. People with a strong internal locus are, generally, less likely to be stressed out than those with an external locus of control. So, the most stressed-out employees are, typically, those who put in long hours for low pay and who exert little control over their working lives, such as people on production-lines, at checkouts and in call centres. While executive stress is fashionable, managers can control their working lives to a much greater extent than their subordinates. INTERHEART found that a high internal locus of control reduced heart attack risk by 32 per cent.

Again, researchers calculated the PAR:

- Stress at home contributed to 8 per cent of first heart attacks.
- Stress at work contributed to 9 per cent.
- Depression contributed to 9 per cent.
- Stressful life events contributed to 10 per cent.
- Financial stress contributed to 11 per cent.
- Stress at both home and work contributed to 12 per cent.
- Low locus of control contributed to 16 per cent.

Some of these overlap. Financial stress can cause depression and problems at home. An external locus of control can contribute to stress at work. After taking the overlaps into account the authors of INTERHEART estimated that stress causes up to a third of heart attacks. In other words, stress and psychological factors are roughly as important as hypertension and obesity as a cause of heart attacks.

Metabolic syndrome

'Metabolic syndrome' describes a cluster of especially influential cardiovascular risk factors. Definitions vary, but if you have at least three of the following, a doctor may diagnose metabolic syndrome:

- A large waistline – abdominal obesity or 'an apple shape' – at least 94 cm in European men and at least 80 cm in European women. Cut-off points differ for certain ethnic origins (see page 106).
- Abnormal lipids, such as low levels of high-density lipoprotein (HDL, see page 34) in your blood or you're taking a medicine (such as a fibrate or niacin – ask your GP or pharmacist if you're not sure) to boost levels of this 'healthy' fat.
- High levels of triglycerides or you're taking medicines to cut levels of this harmful fat.
- Hypertension or you're taking a medicine to reduce your blood pressure.
- Diabetes or a high blood sugar level when you haven't eaten for several hours (an early sign that you may develop diabetes), or you are taking a drug for diabetes.

INTERHEART found that metabolic syndrome increases the risk of the first heart attack by 120 to 169 per cent, depending on the definition used, Mente and colleagues report. The link between the metabolic syndrome and heart attacks was twice as strong in women aged 65 years and younger (361 per cent) as in older women (181 per cent). Metabolic syndrome increases heart attack risk by 166 per cent in men aged 55 years and less and by 119 per cent in older men.

Metabolic syndrome isn't a disease *per se*. But metabolic syndrome reminds us that risk factors for heart attacks commonly cluster. So, if you have one risk factor you should probably ask your GP or nurse to check for others – such as diabetes or hypertension if you're carrying extra weight around your belly. If you've survived a heart attack, you should have been checked – but there's no harm in asking.

Hypertension

As mentioned in Chapter 1, your heart pushes blood along thousands of miles of vessels, which takes considerable force. Blood pressure measures the force exerted against the artery walls. In turn, blood pressure depends on the force generated by the heart, the amount of blood pumped around the circulation, and the size and flexibility of the arteries.

Doctors and nurses measure blood pressure in millimetres of mercury (mmHg) using a sphygmomanometer, introduced by the Italian doctor Scipione Riva-Rocci in 1896. (Physicists originally measured the pressure exerted by fluids by seeing how far a column of mercury moved. The technique for measuring blood pressure has changed. However, the unit of measurement remains the same.) Until recently, doctors and nurses listened for the 'Korotkoff' sounds using a stethoscope. The sound of the blood flowing in the artery changes as the cuff deflates. Today, most use automatic sphygmomanometers.

Doctors and nurses take two readings. For example, assume your blood pressure is 120/80 mmHg. The top reading (120 mmHg) represents the peak systolic pressure as the heart contracts. The bottom reading (80 mmHg) is the lowest diastolic pressure when the heart relaxes between beats. Your blood pressure increases or decreases to meet your body's demands. For example, blood pressure increases when you exercise. However, in some people, blood pressure is excessively high for too long. So, the blood pressure remains elevated when they're just sitting or lying down rather than exercising. Doctors describe dangerously raised blood pressure as 'hypertension'.

In 2011, the National Institute for Health and Clinical Excellence (NICE) made the first major change to hypertension diagnosis for more than a century. NICE now suggests diagnosing hypertension following 24-hour ambulatory blood pressure monitoring (ABPM) rather than a couple of readings in the doctor's surgery. If your blood pressure is 140/90 mmHg or higher when measured by a doctor or nurse, NICE suggests that you wear a device that continually measures your blood pressure over the day. ABPM diagnoses hypertension more accurately, reduces unnecessary treatments and helps avoid white skirt effects (see below).

If you suffer any of the symptoms in Table 3.2, you should see a doctor urgently. These could be a sign of an especially dangerous form of raised blood pressure called malignant hypertension. However, hypertension rarely causes symptoms. So, unless your blood pressure is measured regularly, a stroke or MI may be the first sign you have hypertension.

Table 3.2 Symptoms that could indicate malignant hypertension

Headache – especially if severe

Confusion

Tinnitus, buzzing or noise in the ears

Fatigue

Irregular heartbeat

Nosebleed, without injury

Changes in vision

The hazards of hypertension

Over many years, hypertension can damage arteries, triggering the formation of fatty streaks. Raised blood pressure can also rupture plaques. INTERHEART showed that hypertension roughly doubles MI risk and causes almost a fifth of heart attacks. Indeed, among people aged between 40 and 69 years, each sustained 20 mmHg increase in blood pressure and each sustained 10 mmHg rise in diastolic pressure doubles mortality from heart disease. In people aged 80–89 years, these rises increase the risk of death from heart disease by 50 per cent. Hypertension also contributes to almost three-quarters of strokes.

Antihypertensives – drugs that lower blood pressure – and life-style changes (see Chapter 7) dramatically reduce your risk of suffering a heart attack linked to hypertension. However, while hypertension is one of the most common diseases, it's often poorly treated. In 2008, 32 per cent of men and 29 per cent of women in England had been diagnosed with hypertension. But 53 per cent of men and 41 per cent of women with hypertension were not receiving treatment for raised blood pressure, the BHF comments. Around half of those who were treated remained hypertensive. (These people probably need to take a higher dose or an additional antihypertensive.)

So, you need to take your antihypertensives, change your life-style and monitor your blood pressure regularly. A doctor or nurse should measure your blood pressure at least once a year. You can also buy blood pressure monitors to use at home. However, seek advice first. For example, you need to make sure the monitor is accurate and you have the right-sized cuff. Your GP or hospital, the BHF or the Blood Pressure Association may be able to help.

Strokes

The term 'stroke' conveys the attack's sudden nature: sufferers can fall suddenly to the ground, often senseless, as if they'd been struck by lightning, Pound and co-authors note.

Many strokes are devastating. Around 30 per cent of stroke survivors regain full independence within three weeks, which increases to approximately 50 per cent within six months. However, half of stroke survivors depend on other people for the normal activities of daily living – such as personal hygiene, dressing or eating. Many of those who regain independence after suffering a stroke endure some level of disability.

According to the Stroke Association, about four in every five strokes follow ischaemia, usually after the rupture of a plaque in the arteries supplying the brain. The clot blocks the vessel, thereby starving the brain of oxygen. Fragments of clots elsewhere in the body, air bubbles or fat globules (embolisms) can also travel to and block the arteries supplying the brain. Short-lived blockages in the these arteries can cause transient ischaemic attacks (TIAs), also called mini-strokes. The remainder of strokes (about one in five) occur when a vessel bursts, sending blood flooding into the brain (haemorrhagic stroke).

As the underlying disease is usually the same, many stroke risk factors overlap with those for heart attacks. For example, smoking 20 cigarettes a day increases the likelihood of suffering a stroke six-fold. Drinking large amounts of alcohol and hypertension increase stroke risk three-fold and four-fold, respectively.

The mystery of hypertension

Two per cent of women and 7 per cent of men aged 16–24 years in England are hypertensive. Rates increase to 25 per cent of women and 33 per cent of men aged 45–54 years, and 73 per cent of women and 68 per cent of men aged 75 years or older, the BHF estimate. Why so many people have hypertension is a mystery. Doctors identify an underling cause in only 5–10 per cent of cases – which they call secondary hypertension. Treating secondary hypertension often lowers blood pressure to safe levels.

So, it's worth identifying underlying causes, such as some kidney diseases, Cushing's syndrome (a rare hormonal disease), sleep apnoea, white coat hypertension (see below) and some drugs. Onusko notes that up to 80 per cent of people taking immuno-suppressive drugs and corticosteroids to prevent the body from rejecting an organ transplant show increased blood pressure. Some non-steroidal anti-inflammatory drugs (NSAIDs) – including ibu-profen, naproxen and piroxicam – may raise blood pressure.

Onusko notes that nicotine in cigarettes, smokeless tobacco and cigars raise blood pressure for up to 30 minutes. So, if you can't quit, don't light up just before you go in to have your blood pressure measured. (Nicotine patches do not seem to increase blood pressure.) Drinking excessive amounts of alcohol, eating too much salt and being overweight can also cause secondary hypertension. We'll look at ways to tackle these in Chapter 7.

White coat and white skirt hypertension

Some people have hypertension when the doctor or nurse measures their blood pressure. But outside the clinic, antihypertensives effec-tively control their blood pressure or the pressure is normal. These people have 'white coat hypertension'. The 'stress' of undergoing a medical intervention drives their blood pressure up.

That's one reason why NICE now suggests ABPM before diag-nosing hypertension. For example, Viera and Hinderliter report that around 40 per cent of people taking one or two antihypertensive medicines and almost 30 per cent of those on three medications showed white coat hypertension. So, some of these people may be taking certain medicines unnecessarily.

And it might seem like a joke from *Carry on Doctor*, but Japanese researchers found that when women measured the blood pressure of men aged 18–20 years, diastolic and systolic readings were, on average, 5 mmHg higher than when men made the recording. Almost 11 per cent of young men showed readings sufficient to diagnose isolated systolic hypertension (systolic pressure over 150 mm Hg) when women measured blood pressure compared with 4 per cent when men took the readings. However, the sex of the person measuring did not influence blood pressure or heart rate in females of the same age. The researchers called the phenomenon 'white skirt hypertension'.

Lethal and healthy cholesterol

Some of us lament the end of going to work fuelled by a fry-up. But falling fat consumption has contributed to the decline in deaths from heart disease over the past few years. In 1989, we ate, on average, 112 g of fat a day, the BHF remarks. By 2008, our fat intake had declined to 83 g a day.

Despite its bad press, cholesterol is an essential building block of the membranes surrounding every cell. Cholesterol forms part of the insulation (myelin sheath) around many nerve fibres that ensures that nerve signals travel properly. And cholesterol forms the backbone of several hormones, including oestrogen, testosterone and progesterone. But poor diets and a lack of exercise (which burns up fat) mean that many of us have too much of a good thing.

A common problem

In 2008, about three in every five people in England showed total cholesterol levels that doctors regard as hazardous to the heart's health (5.0 millimoles per litre – mmol/L – or more). A similar proportion of Scottish adults aged 16–64 years showed dangerously raised total cholesterol. Rates of raised cholesterol peak in middle age: more than three-quarters of men aged 45–54 years and women aged 55–64 years have dangerously high levels. Furthermore, one in 14 men and one in 20 women in England have dangerously low levels (less than 1.0 mmol/L) of high-density lipoprotein (HDL) compared with one in six men and one in 17 women in Scotland, the BHF comments.

Transporting cholesterol around the body poses a problem. Blood is about four-fifths water. As oil and water don't mix, your body surrounds a core of fat with soluble coats called lipoproteins. For example:

- Low-density lipoprotein (LDL) carries cholesterol from the liver to the tissues. LDL accumulates in artery walls contributing to atherosclerosis. According to *The Lancet*, each 1.0 mmol/L reduction in LDL reduces deaths by 10 per cent.
- HDL carries between a quarter and a third of blood cholesterol. HDL tends to carry cholesterol away from the arteries and back to the liver for excretion. HDL removes cholesterol from plaques, slowing atherosclerosis.

In other words, high LDL levels increase heart attack risk. High levels of HDL protect against MIs. It's easy to remember: LDL is 'lethal'; HDL is 'healthy'. INTERHEART found that high levels of harmful fats in the blood increased the risk of the first heart attack up to three-fold. So, your doctor will probably measure more than total cholesterol. Your doctor will want to know the balance between HDL and LDL, which may influence treatment (see Chapter 7).

Lipids in INTERHEART

LDL and HDL each contain a different chemical called an apolipoprotein, which helps cells and enzymes recognize and use a specific fat, Walldius and Jungner remark. INTERHEART divided the people that they studied into five groups based on the ratio between the apolipoproteins, which is more precise than measuring HDL and LDL themselves. The coat that surrounds LDL and the other atherogenic (atherosclerosis-causing) fats contains apolipoprotein (apo B). The coat surrounding HDL contains apo A-1. So, increases in apo B and decreases in apo A-1 increase MI risk. Low levels of apo B and increases in apo A-1 reduce the risk. INTERHEART showed that an increase in the ratio (balance) between apoB and ApoA1 can harm your heart. Compared to the lowest ratio, the risk increased between two- and three-fold in those with higher levels.

Triglycerides

Doctors sometimes measure levels of other fats, such as triglycerides and, less commonly, very low density lipoprotein (VLDL). VLDL contains more triglyceride than other lipoproteins. High levels of VLDL or triglyceride increases your risk of coronary artery disease.

Cholesterol and triglycerides are both fats. However, they have very different biological roles. When you eat, your body 'burns' carbohydrates (such as sugar) to meet your immediate energy needs. The body converts any leftover calories into triglycerides, which you store in fat cells. You can then use the energy later. But because we tend to eat regularly, we don't burn the energy stores, and we pile on the pounds.

Lipoproteins rich in triglycerides easily enter damaged artery walls and as they're larger than LDL, they're more likely to remain in the plaque. Once in the plaque, triglycerides trigger inflammation, hinder the breakdown of blood clots and exacerbate the abnormal function of cells lining the artery caused by atherosclerosis.

Several other risk factors, including smoking, type 2 diabetes, obesity and metabolic syndrome increase triglyceride levels. People with high triglyceride levels in their blood tend to have to low levels of HDL, and vice versa. Even allowing for these intimate relationships, raised triglycerides dramatically increase heart attack risk. Kolovou and colleagues report that one study included 13,953 healthy male soldiers aged between 26 and 45 years. Doctors divided the soldiers into five groups based on their triglyceride levels measured after the men hadn't eaten for several hours (the 'fasting level'). After allowing for other risk factors, men with the highest triglyceride levels were about four times more likely to have CHD than those with the lowest.

In another study, men with high non-fasting triglyceride levels (at least 5 mmol/L) were almost five times more likely to suffer heart attacks and around three times more likely to experience ischaemic strokes than those with low levels (less than 1 mmol/L). Women with high triglyceride levels were almost 17 times more likely to experience heart attacks and about five times more likely to suffer ischaemic strokes. So while you're reducing your level of LDL and total cholesterol and boosting your level of HDL, don't neglect triglycerides. Ideally, aim to keep your triglyceride level below 1.7 mmol/L.

Diabetes

Mediaeval doctors regularly inspected their patients' urine by holding a sample in a bulbous glass flask up to the light. Some went further: they took a swig. Indian texts from the fifth century BC and the Islamic philosopher-scientist Avicenna (980–1037) commented that diabetic urine tasted sweet. In 1674, Thomas Willis used the sweet taste to distinguish diabetes from other causes of frequent urination.

Diabetes arises when glucose levels in your blood are too high. A hormone called insulin helps cells take up glucose. The cell then uses glucose to generate energy. If your pancreas does not produce enough insulin, glucose levels in your blood rise to dangerous levels. In other cases, insulin does not work properly (insulin resistance). The body tries to reduce blood glucose levels by flushing the excess out of the body. So, people with diabetes urinate more – and their urine tastes sweet. You should see your doctor if you suffer any symptoms in Table 3.3.

Table 3.3 Common symptoms of diabetes

More frequent urination than usual, especially at night
Increased thirst; drinking excessively
Extreme tiredness and fatigue
Unexplained weight loss
Genital itching or regular episodes of thrush
Cuts and wounds that heal slowly
Blurred vision

Source: Diabetes UK.

Different types of diabetes

Doctors distinguish several types including diabetes insipidus and diabetes mellitus:

- Diabetes insipidus affects only about one in 25,000 people, caused when, for example, infection, injury or drugs, such as lithium used to treat bipolar disorder ('manic depression'), undermine the body's ability to regulate water levels.
- Diabetes mellitus, the type we're interested in, is characterized by excessive levels of glucose (sugar) in the blood. ('Mellitus' means 'honey-sweet' – a reminder of the urine's sugary taste.)

Doctors further subdivide diabetes mellitus into two main types:

- Type 1 diabetes mellitus (previously called insulin-dependent or juvenile diabetes). Our immune system normally distinguishes healthy tissue from invading bacteria or viruses. Occasionally, however, the immune system produces antibodies against healthy tissues (auto-immunity). Rheumatoid arthritis (see below) arises when antibodies attack joints. Similarly, type 1 diabetes arises when antibodies destroy insulin-producing cells in the pancreas. Type 1 diabetes can develop at any age. However, most cases appear before the age of 40 years, and usually in children. According to Diabetes UK, type 1 diabetes accounts for 5–15 per cent of cases.

- Type 2 diabetes mellitus (previously called non-insulin-dependent or adult-onset diabetes) usually occurs in obese and overweight people aged more than 40 years. However, in South Asian and black people, type 2 diabetes typically appears from the age of 25 years. According to Diabetes UK, type 2 diabetes accounts for between 85 and 95 per cent of cases.

As our waistbands expand, more and more of us will develop diabetes. So, increasing numbers of overweight and obese children and adolescents now develop type 2 diabetes. In 2008, doctors diagnosed 145,000 new cases of diabetes, which, Diabetes UK point out, is more than the population of Middlesbrough. In 2009, doctors had diagnosed around 2.6 million people in the UK with diabetes. The charity warns that by 2025, 4.2 million people in the UK will have diabetes.

But many of us have no idea that we've already developed diabetes. Diabetes UK estimates that up to half a million people in the UK have undiagnosed diabetes. So, the first sign that they suffer from diabetes may be a heart attack or another complication, such as nerve pain, an ulcer or changes in vision. Indeed, by the time they're diagnosed, half of people with type 2 diabetes have already developed complications.

Diabetes and heart disease

Type 2 diabetes shortens life expectancy by up to 10 years, largely because of a dramatically increased risk of heart disease. Cardiovascular disease kills 44 per cent of people with type 1 diabetes and 52 per cent with type 2 diabetes, Diabetes UK warns. People with diabetes are also roughly twice as likely to suffer a stroke in the five years after their doctor diagnosed diabetes.

Overall, diabetes increases your risk of suffering CHD between two- and four-fold. Haffner and colleagues found that among people who had not previously suffered a heart attack, approximately 4 per cent of those without diabetes suffered their first MI over the next seven years. This rate was about five times higher in those with diabetes (19 per cent). Diabetes also more than doubled the risk of a further heart attack in those who survived an MI (20 and 45 per cent in those without and with diabetes, respectively).

Moreover, diabetes dramatically cuts your chance of surviving a heart attack. Donahoe and colleagues reported that after allowing for other factors that change CHD risk – such as age, sex, smoking and treatments – death rates following acute coronary syndrome were a third higher among people with diabetes. So, if you have any symptoms in Table 3.3 or you're at high risk (for example, if you're overweight) you should ask your GP to test you for diabetes.

Your heart goes up in smoke

Apart from causing cancer, smoking dramatically increases your risk of suffering a heart attack. According to Action on Smoking and Health (ASH):

- Smoking causes around 25,000 deaths a year from cardiovascular disease.
- Smoking contributes to about one in five premature deaths from heart and circulatory disease.
- Smoking increases the risk of suffering peripheral arterial disease up to four-fold.
- A cigarette smoker is nearly twice as likely to have a heart attack as a non-smoker.

Younger people and women seem to be especially vulnerable to smoking-related heart attacks. Smokers under the age of 40 years are five times more likely to suffer a heart attack than their peers, for example. Grundtvig and colleagues found that smoking lowered the average age that a woman suffered her first heart attack by almost 14 years and by six years among men. As Table 3.4 shows, in women smoking reduced the age of the first heart attack more than suffering from angina or a stroke. In men, the risks associated with smoking, angina and stroke were broadly similar (although that's bad enough!).

Table 3.4 Reduction in the age of first heart attack with smoking, angina and stroke

Risk factor	Reduction in age of first heart attack (years)	
	Women	Men
Smoking	13.7	6.2
Angina before the MI	4.3	6.8
Previously suffered a stroke	4.1	6.9

Based on Grundtvig et al.

Smoking also cuts your chances of surviving an MI. The BHF notes that smokers are 60 per cent more likely to die after they suffer a heart attack than non-smokers. The increased risk rises to 80 per cent among heavy smokers. In another study, people who smoked around the time of their first heart attack were 30 per cent more likely to die in the seven years after their discharge from hospital than non-smokers.

If you don't quit for the sake of your health, think of the heart beating in the chests of your partner or children. Passive smoking accounts for around one in every 100 deaths worldwide, according to Öberg and colleagues. Heart disease causes around 60 per cent of deaths from passive smoking – almost 18 times more than deaths from lung cancer.

So why is smoking so dangerous? Smoking damages the heart in several ways:

- Nicotine triggers adrenaline release. So, the heart beats more rapidly and blood pressure rises. Heart rate begins to rise within a minute of starting to smoke and may increase by up to 30 per cent in the 10 minutes after lighting up.
- Tobacco smoke is rich in carbon monoxide, which reduces the blood's ability to carry oxygen. So, the heart needs to work harder to supply the body with oxygen.
- Smoking increases levels of cholesterol in the blood and undermines the 'balance' between 'healthy' HDL and 'lethal' LDL.
- Smoking increases levels of fibrinogen (a protein that triggers blood clots). So, platelets (blood cells that cause clots) are more likely to clump.

On the other hand, MI risk halves within a year of quitting. People with CHD who quit reduce their risk of dying from the disease by about 40 per cent. Chapter 7 look at ways to quit.

Excess weight and obesity

In the UK, around three-fifths of women and two-thirds of men are overweight or obese. Those extra pounds markedly increase the risk of CHD and heart attacks. Even gaining just 5 kg may, Peters warns, increase CHD risk by 30 per cent. If current trends continue, another 11 million adults in the UK will be obese by 2030, resulting in 331,000 extra cases of CHD and strokes, 545,000 more cases of diabetes and 87,000 additional cancers.

Obesity and several other heart attack risk factors are intimately linked. For example, hypertension is between five and six times more common in obese people (those with a body mass index – BMI – over 30 kg/m^2) compared to those of healthy BMI (18.5–24.9 kg/m^2). Excess weight causes around 90 per cent of cases of type 2 diabetes. Obesity is also a core component of the metabolic syndrome. As a final example: triglycerides store energy in fat cells. Not surprisingly, if your waistband bulges with fat you're likely to have high levels of triglycerides in your blood.

Body mass index (BMI)

Weight itself isn't a very good guide to your risk of developing heart disease and other conditions linked to excess weight. Weighing 90 kg (about 14 stone) is fine if you're 2 metres (about 6 foot 6 inches) tall, but you're seriously obese if you're 1.7 metres (about 5 foot 6 inches). So, BMI assesses whether you're overweight or obese based on your height and weight. BMI estimates, roughly, your amount of body fat and, therefore, your risk of developing diseases linked to excess weight, such as heart disease, hypertension, type 2 diabetes, gallstones, breathing problems and some cancers. You should try to keep your BMI between 18.5 and 24.9 kg/m^2. Below this and you're dangerously underweight. A BMI between 25.0 and 29.9 kg/m^2 suggests that you are overweight. You're probably obese if your BMI exceeds 30.0 kg/m^2. BMI works for most people. However, the BMI may overestimate body fat in athletes, body builders and other muscular people (such as hod carriers). On the other hand, BMI may underestimate body fat in older persons and others who have lost muscle. You doctor can check your body fat level using a special monitor.

Triglycerides and obesity

The EPIC–Norfolk study found that a man aged between 45 and 79 years with a waist circumference of at least 90 cm *and* a triglyceride level of at least 2.0 mmol/L was about two and a half times more likely to develop coronary artery disease over the decade-long study than those below these values. A woman with a waist circumference of at least 85 cm *and* a triglyceride level of at least 1.5 mmol/L was almost four times more likely to develop coronary artery disease. Similarly, Lemieux and colleagues found that a man with a waist circumference of less than 90 cm and a triglyceride level of at least 2.0 mmol/L was two and a half times more likely to show a plaque that blocked more than half of a major coronary artery. A man with this level of triglyceride and a waist circumference of at least 90 cm was almost four times more likely to show such a severely blocked vessel.

More than blubber

Doctors traditionally believed that obesity increased the likelihood of suffering a heart attack because fat acted as a 'marker' for other risk factors, such as hypertension and increased cholesterol levels. These two influences account for about 45 per cent of the increased risk of CHD in overweight people. But we now know that, far from being inert blubber, fat (which biologists call adipose tissue) is a biological factory continuously pumping out chemicals, including messengers called adipokines. That's one reason why being overweight – even moderately overweight – increases CHD risk independently of blood pressure and cholesterol.

Broadly, the body produces two types of fat. A layer of subcutaneous fat just below the skin conserves body heat. Abdominal (visceral) fat is more active than the subcutaneous layer, pumping out adipokines, some of which increase inflammation. In turn, inflammation promotes atherosclerosis and damages blood vessels. Logue and colleagues found that, after other risk factors were allowed for, obesity increased the risk of fatal heart disease between 60 and 75 per cent. Similarly, Coutinho and colleagues found that in people with coronary artery disease, central obesity increased mortality by 70 per cent *even in people with a healthy BMI*. The increased risk of death reached 93 per cent in obese people. So, try to maintain a healthy BMI (18.5–24.9 kg/m^2) – especially if you carry the excess pounds around your waist.

Other cardiovascular risk factors

Over the years, doctors linked up to 300 risk factors to heart disease and MIs. Many more are emerging as doctors examine the impact of genes. There's not space here to look at all of these. However, the following are worth mentioning, largely because you and your doctor can take steps to reduce the risk.

For example, persistently raised heart rate – even if not severe enough to be an arrhythmia – increases the risk of cardiovascular disease and death to a similar degree as smoking, raised cholesterol and hypertension. Kannel and co-workers found that in people with untreated hypertension, each rise in heart rate of 40 bpm increased mortality from cardiovascular disease, including coronary artery disease, by approximately 70 per cent. Deaths from any cause approximately doubled. On the other hand, regular exercise reduces heart rate.

Early heart attacks

Genes rather than lifestyle sometimes raise cholesterol to dangerous levels. Around 120,000 people in Britain suffer from familial hypercholesterolaemia (FH), an inherited disorder that causes high blood cholesterol from birth. So, a person with FH often suffers a heart attack relatively young. Yet 85 per cent of those affected don't know they have FH, which is caused by an abnormal gene that produces a protein (the LDL receptor) that removes LDL from the blood. Several other less common genetic disorders also increase blood cholesterol levels.

Chronic kidney disease

In the UK, diabetes and hypertension are the leading causes of chronic kidney disease, which affects about one in 13 of the population. People with diabetes attempt to normalize blood glucose levels by excreting sugar in urine. But this can damage their kidneys. Similarly, hypertension can damage blood vessels in the kidneys. So, diabetes and hypertension undermine the kidneys' ability to excrete waste and superfluous fluid. The extra fluid stays in the circulation, pushing blood pressure higher. Unless hypertension or diabetes is treated, the cycle of damage may leave the person needing a kidney transplant or dialysis.

Most of us are born with more kidney function than we need. Indeed 'living donors' can live healthy and full lives despite donating a kidney. This 'reserve' means that mild chronic kidney disease doesn't cause symptoms and often remains undiagnosed. As a result, up to one in 10 of us could suffer from kidney disease. However, as kidney disease progresses you may develop symptoms including: tiredness; swollen ankles, feet or hands caused by water retention; shortness of breath; itchy skin; nausea; and, in men, problems having or keeping an erection. You should see your doctor if you develop any of these symptoms.

Chronic kidney disease markedly increases heart attack risk. Meisinger and colleagues found that in women aged 45–74 years chronic kidney disease increased the risk of suffering a heart attack by 67 per cent and the risk of cardiovascular death by 60 per cent. In men, the increased risks were 51 and 48 per cent, respectively. Indeed, chronic kidney disease may be more hazardous to your heart than diabetes. In a decade-long study, Debella and colleagues found that after allowing for other risk factors, people with chronic kidney disease were 3.5 times more likely to suffer a heart attack than those with healthy kidneys. This compared to a 2.5-fold increase among those with diabetes.

If you have kidney disease you begin to excrete protein in your urine: a condition called albuminuria or proteinuria. Using a dip-stick to test for small increases in levels of albumin – the commonest protein in blood – in the urine (microalbuminuria) can identify early kidney disease long before you develop symptoms. Certain drugs – including angiotensin converting enzyme (ACE) inhibitors and angiotensin receptor antagonists (see Chapter 5) – seem to slow the progression of kidney disease. So it's worth checking whether you've been tested recently.

Gout

Few diseases match the pain caused by gout. The Reverend Sydney Smith, a nineteenth-century wit, described his attacks as like 'walking on eyeballs'. Gout left the eminent seventeenth-century physician Thomas Sydenham unable to endure 'the shaking of the room from a person's walking briskly therein'. Far from being a historical curiosity, gout remains the most common inflammatory joint disease among men older than 40 years of age. When my father suffered an acute attack of gout, he had to sleep with his foot poking from underneath the bedclothes. He couldn't even bear the sheets touching his big toe.

Gout occurs when crystals of sodium urate – the salt of uric acid – deposit in the joints. In turn, uric acid forms when the body breaks down chemicals called purines, which are found in, for example, offal DNA (which carries your genetic code) and caffeine. Acute gout typically develops rapidly, often beginning at night and usually affecting a single joint. Roddy points out that the ancient Greeks called the disease *podagra* – 'foot-grabber' – reflecting that, in up to around three-quarters of cases, gout initially arises in the toe joints.

Numerous CHD risk factors increase the likelihood of developing gout. For example, according to Soriano and colleagues:

- People who drank between 25 and 42 units of alcohol a week were 145 per cent more likely to develop gout than abstainers. The risk increased to 200 per cent among those drinking more than 42 units per week.
- Overweight people were 62 per cent more likely to develop gout than those with a BMI in the healthy range. The risk increased to 134 per cent among the obese.
- Chronic kidney disease (148 per cent increase), heart failure (84 per cent), ischaemic heart disease (19 per cent), hypertension (18 per cent) all increase gout risk.
- Raised levels of triglycerides (45 per cent increase) or cholesterol (8 per cent) and other dyslipidaemias (21 per cent) increased the chances of developing gout.
- Psoriasis (see below) increased the risk of gout by 12 per cent.

This overlap means that if you suffer from gout it's probably worth asking your doctor or nurse to check if you have hypertension, an abnormal lipid profile, diabetes or kidney disease.

Inflammatory diseases: psoriasis and rheumatoid arthritis

Around one person in every 50 in the UK suffers from psoriasis: red, flaky, crusty patches of skin covered with silvery scales. (Psoriasis is not infectious. Nevertheless, people with psoriasis often experience unjustified prejudice, such as being asked to leave swimming pools and changing rooms in shops.)

The inflammation that causes psoriasis can spill out from the skin, causing problems elsewhere in the body, including worsening your prospects following a heart attack. Ahlehoff and colleagues found that in the approximately 21 months after suffering their first MI, people with psoriasis were 18 per cent to die than heart attack survivors without the skin disease. The risk of another heart attack, stroke and death from cardiovascular disease together was 26 per cent higher among those with psoriasis.

Around 400,000 people in the UK endure the distress, discomfort and disability arising from rheumatoid arthritis, which shortens life expectancy by about 10 years. For example, Meune and colleagues reported that rheumatoid arthritis increased the risk of fatal stokes by 46 per cent, fatal heart attacks by 77 per cent, all strokes (fatal and non-fatal) by 91 per cent and all MIs by 110 per cent. Holmqvist and collaborators found that people with rheumatoid arthritis were 60 per cent more likely to suffer a heart attack than those without the joint disease.

In both psoriasis and rheumatoid arthritis, increased inflammation seems to be responsible for the rise in heart disease risk. So, it's important to discuss the most effective way of tackling these diseases with your GP or specialist. In some cases, the doctor may suggest more 'aggressive' heart disease prevention with drugs, in line with your increased risk.

4

Diagnosing heart attacks

Despite being one of the most common diseases, even experienced doctors find some heart attacks surprisingly difficult to diagnose. Typically, the lack of oxygen to the heart causes pain or discomfort in the chest, abdomen, wrist or jaw, according to Alpert and colleagues. However, not everyone develops these classic 'ischaemic' symptoms and, as this chapter shows, doctors use several techniques to determine whether you've suffered a heart attack. While symptoms can differ, early treatment offers your best chance of surviving an MI: if in doubt call 999.

Symptoms of a heart attack

Despite their variability, the pattern of symptoms offers an important clue. For example, the discomfort caused by a heart attack can occur with or without exertion and does not usually go away with rest. In contrast, exertion or emotions tend to trigger stable angina, which subsides on rest. In general, the pain of a heart attack is more persistent that the pain of stable angina. For instance, around 80 per cent of people with unstable angina or a related type of heart attack called a NSTEMI (see page 53) experience chest pain that lasts more than 20 minutes. Nevertheless, these aren't hard-and-fast rules: in some heart attacks the pain is short-lived.

Most people report that the pain or discomfort caused by a heart attack begins in the centre or left side of their chest, then radiates to the arm, jaw, back or shoulder. The pain isn't usually 'sharp' and tends to be diffuse rather than confined to a small area. Heart attacks may trigger breathlessness, heavy sweating, nausea, vomiting or light-headedness. Moving the muscles around the site of the discomfort, taking a deep breath or changing position doesn't usually affect the pain.

Alan's story

For the past two years, Alan, a 54-year-old electrician, suffered angina when he worked especially hard – such as doing heavy digging. So, he was surprised when he suffered an angina attack walking home from the local shops. He sprayed his glyeryl trinitrate (GTN) into his mouth and dismissed the attack as 'just one of those things'. (GTN opens the heart's blood vessels and so alleviates angina.) He didn't tell his wife – 'she'd just worry'. However, two days later he suffered another attack while changing a light bulb. The first GTN dose didn't help. But the second dose alleviated the pain. Later that evening he suffered angina while he was watching television. This time the second spray didn't work. His wife – barely containing her anger because he'd kept the previous attacks quiet – gave him an aspirin to chew and phoned the ambulance. Alan had suffered his first heart attack. He recovered fully and nine weeks later was back at work.

The popular idea of a heart attack is a grimacing man suddenly gripping his chest. But around two-thirds of people experience symptoms, including shortness of breath and fatigue, in the days to weeks before they suffer an MI. In many cases, stable angina suddenly becomes more frequent or more severe, lasts for longer or is provoked by less intense activity – a condition called 'crescendo angina'. So, you need to remain alert for possible warning signs, such as a change in your pattern of angina, and see your GP as soon as possible.

When to call 999

If you suffer chest pain or other symptoms that you think could mean you're suffering a heart attack *and* your doctor has diagnosed angina, stop what you are doing, sit down and rest. Take your GTN spray or tablets. If the pain doesn't ease within five minutes, take your GTN again. If the pain does not ease within five minutes of taking the second dose of GTN, call 999 immediately.

If you haven't been diagnosed with angina (or you don't have your medicine) and suffer symptoms that could suggest a heart attack, sit down and rest. If the pain doesn't go away in a couple of minutes, you should call 999 for an ambulance. Even if the pain resolves, you should see your GP as soon as you can.

> If you're not allergic to aspirin and you don't suffer from aspirin-sensitive asthma, chew an adult aspirin tablet (300 mg) if there is one to hand or someone can get the tablet for you. It might be worth carrying some aspirin tablets with you. If you can't reach the aspirin easily, or you are allergic to aspirin, the BHF suggests resting until the ambulance arrives. Remember, the symptoms of a heart attack can vary – so if you're worried call 999 immediately.

Atypical symptoms

Many heart attack victims report 'atypical' symptoms. During a heart attack, some people develop pain in their upper abdomen, which patients and doctors may confuse with indigestion. Other people having an MI suffer pain in their arm, shoulder, wrist, jaw or back without experiencing chest discomfort. According to the Royal College of Psychiatrists, around a quarter of people who go to an A&E department with chest pain are having a panic attack rather than a heart attack. (But don't assume it's anxiety: it could prove a fatal mistake.)

Atypical heart attacks are especially common in younger people (those aged 25–40 years) and older people (those aged over 75 years), in women and in those with diabetes, chronic kidney disease, dementia, unstable angina or a NSTEMI (see page 53). For instance, people with unstable angina or a NSTEMI may report: abdominal pain; bouts of indigestion; sharp stabbing chest pain, which may be worse when they breathe in; and increasing breathlessness. Bassand and colleagues comment that the absence of the classic chest pain in many people with unstable angina and NSTEMI means that these conditions often remain undiagnosed and inadequately treated.

In other words, doctors can't rely on symptoms alone to diagnose heart attacks. So, they use a variety of tests and consider the results together. According to Alpert and colleagues, doctors diagnose a heart attack based on characteristic changes in levels of enzymes released into your blood (see below) as well as one the following:

- symptoms of ischaemia – such as chest pain;
- new Q waves on ECG (see below);
- ECG changes indicating ischaemia (see below);

- Needing heart surgery – such as angioplasty (see Chapter 5) – to reopen blocked coronary blood vessels during that admission to hospital.

In addition, doctors may use imaging techniques (see below) to locate the blocked coronary artery. However, imaging isn't needed to diagnose a heart attack. Each test adds a piece to the jigsaw that leads the doctor to diagnose a MI or unstable angina (Table 4.1).

Table 4.1 Features of heart attack revealed by different tests

Test	Feature
Examination of heart tissue under the microscope	Death of heart cells
Blood tests	Markers of damage to the heart – e.g. CK-MB and cardiac troponins T and I
Electrocardiography	Changes in the ST–T segment may indicate ischaemia
	Q waves, suggesting loss of electrically normal heart tissue
Imaging	Reduced or lost blood supply to the heart
	Abnormal motion of the heart wall

Based on Alpert et al.

Blood markers

Blood tests are the keystone of the diagnosis of a heart attack. During an MI, oxygen starvation caused by the blocked coronary artery gradually kills the area of heart muscle supplied by that vessel. Alpert and colleagues note that the death of the entire vulnerable area takes at least four to six hours, depending on the extent of the blood supply from other vessels, whether the blockage is persistent or intermittent, and the sensitivity of the muscle. Over this time, damaged heart muscles release a cocktail of proteins into the blood, which aid diagnosis:

- Myoglobin: a protein that binds oxygen in muscle, similar to the way that haemoglobin binds oxygen in red blood cells. Myoglobin provides extra oxygen, allowing muscles to remain active for longer. Levels of myoglobin can rise following damage to several types of muscle, and so are not specific for heart damage.

- Lactate dehydrogenase, an enzyme that helps keep cells supplied with energy when oxygen is limited. Levels rise following damage to several types of muscle.
- Creatine kinase, another enzyme involved in supplying cells with energy. The body produces three types of creatine kinase. One of these – creatine kinase MB (CK-MB) – comes mainly, but not solely, from the heart. So, CK-MB levels usually rise only following damage to heart muscles. However, CK-MB is not as specific for the heart muscle as cardiac troponins T and I.

Measuring levels of cardiac troponins T and I is the best way for doctors to assess damage to your heart muscle. Troponins are specialized proteins that help muscles contract. The specific type of troponin depends on the muscle. The heart accounts for almost all the body's production of cardiac troponin I and T. So, these proteins are very sensitive markers of damage to heart muscle. For instance, doctors use cardiac troponins T and I to distinguish unstable angina (when levels don't rise) from a heart attack.

Nevertheless, Alpert and colleagues note, while a rise in CK-MB or cardiac troponins T and I, or both, means that the heart muscle has been damaged, the tests don't reveal *how* the damage occurred. So, if a doctor finds raised levels of cardiac troponins T and I, but you haven't experienced ischaemic symptoms (such as angina), the doctor will look for other causes, such as myocarditis (inflammation of heart muscle), before concluding that you've suffered an MI.

Electrocardiogram (ECG)

As we saw in Chapter 1, a wave of electrical activity spreads across the heart so that the atria and ventricles contract in the correct sequence. ECGs, introduced in 1901 by Willem Einthoven, measure this electrical activity and record your heart rate, which offer doctors a window through which they can assess your heart's health. So, apart from helping to diagnose MIs, ECGs can:

- detect problems with heart rhythm, such as atrial fibrillation (see Chapter 6);
- distinguish two important subtypes of MI (see below);
- indicate the cause of, or changes produced by, heart failure.

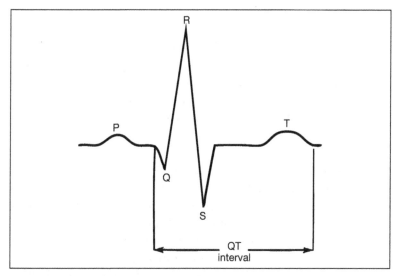

Figure 4.1 A typical ECG in a healthy person

During an ECG, the doctor, nurse or technician sticks small 'electrodes' on to the skin of your arms, legs and chest. They connect the electrodes to an ECG machine, which detects the electrical signals and shows the results on a piece of paper or, more commonly, on a screen. An ECG takes only a few minutes and is painless.

As Figure 4.1 shows, an ECG has several components (see Chapter 1 if you need to remind yourself about the heart's electrical conducting system):

- When the sinoatrial node fires, the electrical wave stimulates both atria, creating the P wave.
- The QRS complex reflects the movement of the impulse from the bundle of His and across the right and left ventricles. Because the ventricles are more muscular than the atria, the QRS complex is larger than the P wave.
- The T wave shows the recovery of the ventricles ready for the next contraction. Essentially, the T wave is the time between heartbeats.

Doctors sometimes look at other measurements. For example:

- A prolonged QT interval – the beginning of the QRS complex to the end of the T wave – is a risk factor for ventricular arrhythmias and sudden death.

- Some heart attacks produce Q waves, which reflect an absence of electrical activity in dead muscle. As mentioned above, the damage to the heart takes hours or days to evolve fully. So, Q waves usually emerge several hours to days after a heart attack, although not all MI survivors show this characteristic change.

Types of ECG

Usually, you'll have your ECG taken while lying down – such as in the doctor's surgery, in A&E or on the hospital ward. However, in some cases, your doctor may monitor your heart continuously as you get on with your usual life over 24 hours (an ambulatory ECG or Holter monitoring). This can detect problems, such as bouts of atrial fibrillation, that only occur from time to time. Electrodes taped to your chest attach to a recorder worn around your waist.

If the symptoms are even less frequent, the doctor may use a 'cardiac event recorder' to record the heart's activity for longer or when symptoms occur. In some cases, you hold the recorder to your chest when you suffer a symptom. Doctors may insert an implantable loop recorder under your skin, which monitors your heart continuously for up to 14 months.

Your doctor might use an ECG to monitor your heart while you walk on a treadmill or pedal a stationary bike. This 'stress' or 'exercise tolerance' test sees how well your heart works during activity. You'll begin at an easy pace and gradually increase the intensity of exercise. The doctor, nurse or technician will monitor your ECG regularly during the test, which usually lasts for up to 15 minutes. You should tell the doctor, nurse or technician if you develop chest pain or discomfort, experience other symptoms or become very tired or breathless.

ST-segment elevation

Alpert and colleagues point out that the death of heart muscle does not always cause ECG abnormalities. In other words, a normal ECG does not rule out a heart attack. Nevertheless, ECGs offer some important diagnostic clues. As we've seen, some heart attacks produce Q waves, while changes to the ST segment help distinguish different types of heart attack.

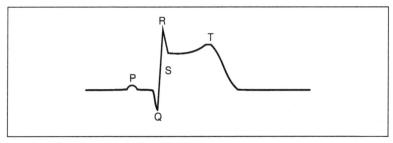

Figure 4.2 ST-segment elevation

Usually, the ST segment, which connects the QRS complex and the T wave, shows a slight concave rise. Ischaemia during exercise, angina and some heart attacks can produce a flat, downward sloping or depressed ST segment. In contrast, up to about half of heart attacks – usually when the clot completely blocks the vessel – produce abnormal elevation of the ST segment (Figure 4.2). So, doctors separate heart attacks into:

- ST-segment elevation MI (STEMI); and
- non-ST-segment elevation MI (NSTEMI).

Like NSTEMI, unstable angina does not elevate the ST-segment. However, in NSTEMI, damage to the heart muscle triggers the release of markers, such as cardiac troponins. These markers don't rise in unstable angina.

These differences in the ST segment are of more than academic interest. Some studies suggest that death while in hospital is more common following STEMI (7 per cent) than with unstable angina and NSTEMI (5 per cent). Death rates were similar after 6 months (12 per cent and 13 per cent, respectively). But after four years, people with unstable angina or NSTEMI were twice as likely to have died than those with STEMI, Bassand and colleagues note. Furthermore, despite modern treatments, about 30 per cent of people with unstable angina suffer another 'adverse outcome' over the next six months, such as death, non-fatal heart attack, angina or another admission for unstable angina.

Unstable angina and NSTEMI tend to occur in people with more extensive disease in their coronary arteries. Those who suffer unstable angina and NSTEMI also tend to be older and more commonly suffer other ailments, especially kidney disease and diabetes. So, the poorer long-term prospects are perhaps not surprising.

NSTEMI and diabetes

Donahoe and colleagues found that 22 per cent of people with unstable angina or NSTEMI had diabetes, compared with 15 per cent of those with STEMI. Among those with unstable angina or NSTEMI, people with diabetes were more likely than those without diabetes to die over the next 30 days (2 per cent and 1 per cent, respectively) and during the first year (7 per cent and 3 per cent, respectively) than those without diabetes. Even allowing for other risk factors, diabetics with unstable angina and NSTEMI were 78 per cent more likely than non-diabetics to die after 30 days and 65 per cent more likely to die after a year.

Imaging and angiography

Your doctor may suggest cardiac imaging using one of two main methods:

- Echocardiograms use high-frequency sound waves (ultrasound) to examine your heart, reveal blockages in your coronary circulation and evaluate your heart valves. You can undergo an echocardiogram while exercising on a treadmill.
- Nuclear cardiac imaging uses a small amount of radioactive material (a tracer or radionuclide) to diagnose coronary artery disease. While there is no 'safe' level of radiation, most doctors believe that the benefits far outweigh the risk associated with the tiny dose of radiation. If you're worried, talk to your doctor or radiographer.

Cardiac imaging can help detect a heart attack or ischaemia as well as identifying other conditions that cause chest pain. Cardiac imaging can also predict your short- and long-term prognosis as well as detecting some complications following a heart attack. However, the damage needs to be relatively extensive before cardiac imaging can detect the problem. For example:

- At least 20 per cent of the thickness of the myocardial wall needs to be damaged before echocardiography can detect abnormal movements of the wall.

- At least 10 g of myocardial tissue (an average heart weighs between 200 and 300 g) needs to be damaged before a radionuclide can detect the injury.

Neither echocardiogram nor nuclear cardiac imaging can distinguish ischaemia from an MI.

Angiography

In 1895, the German scientist Wilhelm Conrad Roentgen was experimenting with vacuum tubes. By accident, he discovered X-rays and, a week later, took the first radiograph – of his wife's hand showing her bones and wedding ring. Bones and teeth are denser than skin. So, they absorb more X-rays than other tissues. As a result, the X-ray film or, more commonly today, detectors show bones as silhouettes.

Coronary arteries aren't dense enough to show up on X-rays. So, during 'angiography', the radiographer injects 'contrast medium' into your coronary arteries using a catheter (a thin, flexible, hollow tube). The contrast medium absorbs X-rays and, therefore, reveals the arteries and their smaller branches. Blood should flow freely around the coronary circulation spreading the contrast media around the blood vessels. So, the X-ray image (angiogram) can show the site and severity of any narrowing in the coronary arteries. This helps the doctor decide the best treatment. For example, a marked narrowing may need bypass surgery or coronary angioplasty, treatments discussed in Chapter 5.

5

Treating heart attacks

As we've seen, MIs strike when the oxygen supply to the heart fails, usually when a clot blocks one or more coronary arteries. So, treating a heart attack aims to restore blood flow through the blocked arteries, keep the vessels open and improve the supply of nutrients and oxygen to the damaged area. Doctors call this 'reperfusion'. It's a bit like unblocking a drain, with a chemical (drugs) or a rod (surgery).

The sooner reperfusion begins, the better your chances of survival. More than half the people who die from MIs within 30 days of suffering a heart attack succumb before medical assistance arrives or they reach hospital. Approximately a third of deaths from a heart attack occur within an hour of symptoms emerging, usually because of a fatal arrhythmia. The longer the delay between symptoms and doctors and your body's clot-busting defences establishing reperfusion, the greater the damage to your heart and the lower your chances of survival. This chapter focuses on the ways doctors unblock the coronary vessels and the other treatments that bolster your chances. However, the exact treatment depends on your particular circumstances. So, the details may vary.

What can I expect?

The immediate aim of paramedics and doctors is to alleviate pain. In the ambulance, you may inhale oxygen or a mixture of nitrous oxide and oxygen (Entonox). The paramedics may offer other painkillers (analgesics) if you are in severe discomfort and, if you've not taken one already, an aspirin to chew.

Once you reach A&E, a doctor or cardiac nurse specialist will assess your symptoms, record your medical history, measure your blood pressure and heart rate, perform an ECG and take a blood sample, such as to measure cardiac troponins T and I (see Chapter

4). Meanwhile, they'll aim to relieve symptoms and reduce the damage to your heart. So, you may receive:

- Aspirin (if you've not received it previously).
- Oxygen – increasing the oxygen level in your blood means that your heart doesn't have to work as hard.
- Morphine, which remains the most effective painkiller. You almost certainly won't become addicted to morphine used to relieve the pain of a heart attack.
- A nitrate injected into your vein, which opens coronary arteries and increases blood flow to the heart. (The technical term for this type of drug is a vasodilator.) So, nitrates relieve chest pain and reduce heart damage. Perez and colleagues found that starting nitrates within 24 hours of a heart attack beginning prevented one death during the first 2 days after an MI for every 125 to 250 people treated. You may receive other vasodilators, such as beta-blockers and ACE inhibitors.
- Thrombolysis or coronary angioplasty with stents (see page 68).

Meanwhile, a heart monitor will check for arrhythmias. You may also undergo other tests – such as a chest X-ray, echocardiogram, exercise ECG, nuclear cardiac imaging or magnetic resonance imaging (MRI) scan and coronary angiography – depending on your history and symptoms.

What happens next depends on the results of these investigations. For example:

- If tests and symptoms suggest that a blood clot has blocked a coronary artery *and* the troponin test results are positive, the doctor will probably tell you that you've suffered a heart attack. In this case, you may receive heparin, a glycoprotein IIb/IIIa inhibitor, a nitrate, a beta-blocker and an ACE inhibitor.
- If the troponin test results are negative, the doctor will probably tell you that you have unstable angina. You may receive heparin, a nitrate and a beta-blocker.

You may receive other drugs if there is a medical reason why you can't receive one of these medcines or you suffer from another problem as well.

Drugs made an important contribution to the decline in deaths from heart disease in recent years. Unal and colleagues estimated that deaths from CHD in England and Wales among men and women aged 35 to 84 years old decreased by 62 per cent and 45 per cent, respectively, between 1981 and 2000. Reduced smoking accounted for 48 per cent of the decline. Improved drugs and surgery accounted for 42 per cent. Over the next few pages, we'll look at some of the drugs used to treat heart attacks.

Aspirin

Aspirin is part of a medical tradition stretching back thousands of years. Plants evolved a chemical called salicylic acid as part of their defences against disease. Our ancestors learnt that consuming plants containing salicylates alleviated pain, inflammation and fever. For example, the Ebers Papyrus, an Egyptian text written some 3,500 years ago, suggests using herbal painkillers that we now know contain salicylates. Greek and Roman healers employed salicylate-containing plants to alleviate rheumatism.

Traditional British healers used willow bark, which is rich in salicylic acid, to alleviate pain and fever. In 1763, Edward Stone, a vicar in the Oxfordshire village of Chipping Norton, found that a dram (about 1.8 g) of willow bark extract alleviated fever. Then in 1827, a French scientist isolated a chemical called salicin from the meadowsweet. German chemists synthesized salicylic acid, a derivative of salicin, in 1860, followed by another chemical variation, acetylsalicylic acid, in 1899, marketed as Aspirin. The brand name Aspirin commemorates the meadowsweet, which then had the Latin name *Spiraea ulmaria*. (Botanists later remained meadowsweet *Filipendula ulmaria*.) Today, their chemical offspring – drugs called non-steroidal anti-inflammatory drugs (NSAIDs), which include ibuprofen, diclofenac and naproxen – are among the most widely prescribed medicines.

In 1948 Lawrence Craven, a GP in California, reported that none of 400 men to whom he had prescribed daily aspirin suffered heart attacks over two years. He suggested, Miner and Hoffhines comment, that men might avoid 'dying a horribly painful death if they would take a couple of aspirins daily for the rest of their lives'. However, few doctors noticed his papers. Then in 1989, the Physicians' Health Study showed that aspirin cuts the risk of heart attacks. Several other studies confirmed the results and suggested that aspirin reduces the risk of death by up to 23 per cent if you start taking it when you first suspect a heart attack and then for the next 30 days.

How aspirin works

Aspirin targets small, irregularly shaped blood cells called platelets. When you start bleeding, platelets gather at the wound and stick together forming a clot. Plaque rupture triggers platelets to clump inside the vessel. Aspirin prevents platelet aggregation by reducing production of a chemical called thromboxane.

Prostaglandins and thromboxane

In the 1930s, the Swedish scientist Ulf von Euler discovered that sperm contained a substance that made the womb contract. von Euler believed that the prostate gland made the substance, which he named prostaglandin. We now know that cells throughout the body make numerous prostaglandins, which carry messages between neighbouring cells. Some prostaglandins trigger pain and inflammation. Cells make thromboxane from one particular prostaglandin.

Thromboxane activates new platelets, enhances platelet aggregation and encourages blood clots. Aspirin blocks the cell's ability to produce thromboxane and so reduces clot formation. (Specifically, aspirin blocks the enzyme, called cyclo-oxygenase, that controls prostaglandin production.) So, you should never take aspirin – to relieve a headache for example – if you're using other anticoagulants (see below) unless your doctor suggests the combination. You could risk excessive bleeding and even a haemorrhagic stroke.

Once you're discharged after your heart attack, your doctor will probably suggest that you take a low-dose aspirin (probably 75 mg) every day to reduce your chance of suffering another MI (secondary prevention). Doctors may also prescribe low-dose aspirin if you haven't suffered acute coronary syndrome (primary prevention) if you're at particularly high risk. They might suggest another anti-platelet drug if you can't take aspirin.

Despite the benefits, around half of people stop taking aspirin. It's a dangerous decision. García Rodríguez and colleagues remark that people who stopped taking aspirin after an MI were 63 per cent more likely to suffer another non-fatal heart attack. Overall, people who stopped their aspirin were 43 per cent more likely either to suffer a non-fatal heart attack or to die from CHD. So you need to keep taking your aspirin. (See page 115 for some tips to ensure you don't forget to take your drugs.)

ACE inhibitors

As we've seen, kidney disease contributes to heart attacks. The kidneys help to control the amount of fluid you excrete in your urine and, in turn, to control your blood pressure. Several chemicals interact to control kidney function. For example, aldosterone tells your kidneys to excrete less water. This increases blood volume, driving blood pressure up. To understand how ACE inhibitors work, we need to follow this pathway backwards.

A protein called angiotensin II triggers aldosterone release from your adrenal glands, which sit on top of your kidneys. Angiotensin II also narrows blood vessels, which increases blood pressure. In turn, an enzyme called ACE (angiotensin converting enzyme) converts a relatively inactive protein called angiotensin I into angiotensin II (Figure 5.1). So, blocking ACE reduces levels of angiotensin II and blood pressure declines. That's how ACE inhibitors – drugs such as captopril, enalapril and lisinopril – work.

ACE inhibitors improve your chances of surviving a heart attack. Starting ACE inhibitors within 24 hours of a heart attack improved

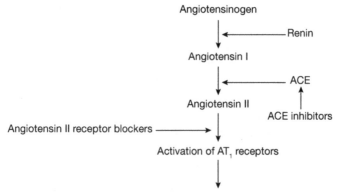

Figure 5.1 How ACE inhibitors work

survival by 7 per cent compared with an inactive placebo (see page 109) over (in most of the 18 studies analysed) five to six weeks. The benefits of ACE inhibitors were most marked in people who had heart failure and a related condition called left ventricular systolic dysfunction (see Chapter 6). In these cases, ACE inhibitors increased survival after an MI by 26 per cent compared with placebo, NICE reports.

Some people benefit from longer-term treatment with ACE inhibitors. An analysis of six trials examined people with stable coronary artery disease whose left ventricles worked normally. (We'll see why this matters in Chapter 6.) Over an average of 4.4 years, ACE inhibitors reduced cardiovascular deaths by 17 per cent, the number of non-fatal heart attacks by 16 per cent, all-cause mortality by 13 per cent and the need for coronary revascularization surgery (see below) by 7 per cent, Perez and colleagues found. After ten days, ACE inhibitors prevented one death in every 200 to 333 people treated.

How some drugs work: a brief aside

Understanding how some other drugs used to treat heart attacks work means taking a brief diversion. Numerous chemicals pass messages around your body. For example:

- Hormones (such as oestrogen, testosterone and aldosterone) carry signals between organs – such as from a gland to fat cells, the kidney and the heart.
- Adipokines carry messages between fat and other cells, such as to promote inflammation and control appetite.
- Neurotransmitters pass messages between nerves as well as between nerves and muscles. For example, noradrenaline increases the force and rate at which the heart contracts. Acetylcholine has the opposite effect. The balance between the two neurotransmitters allows the heart to match its activity to your body's needs.

Many messengers act by binding to specific proteins, called receptors. Imagine a heart muscle cell as a car. The receptor is the ignition lock. The messenger – such as noradrenaline or acetylcholine – is the key. When the key fits into a lock, the engine starts (Figure 5.2). When the messenger binds to the receptor, part of the cell's internal

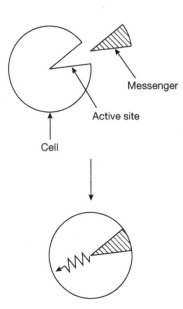

Messenger

Active site

Cell

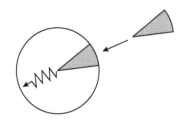

Agonists bind to the active site and trigger the messages, producing the same biological effect as the messenger or neurotransmitter

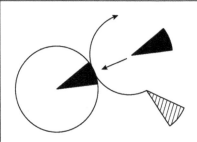

The neurotransmitter or another messenger binds to the active site triggering the messages inside the cell that produce the biological effect

Antagonists bind to the active site and don't trigger the messages, but they prevent the messenger from binding, so blocking the biological effect

Figure 5.2 Drugs and receptors

machine starts. For example, angiotensin II narrows blood vessels and triggers aldosterone release by binding to a receptor known as AT_1 (see Figure 5.1). This binding is specific: your key starts only your car. Noradrenaline doesn't bind to the receptor for acetylcholine or vice versa.

Now imagine you have a skeleton key. It also fits the ignition lock and switches on the engine. Some drugs act like a skeleton key. The receptor can't distinguish the drug (called an agonist) from the normal messenger. Both switch on the cell's machinery. For example, adrenaline, which treats cardiac arrest, binds to and stimulates noradrenaline receptors (see Figure 5.2).

Imagine you have another key. It fits the ignition lock, but won't turn. So, the car won't start. But while this key is in the lock, you can't get the right key in. Some drugs bind to the receptor but don't activate the internal machinery (see Figure 5.2). These are antagonists or 'blockers'. Angiotensin II receptor blockers, used to treat hypertension and heart failure, prevent angiotensin II from binding to AT_1 receptors (see Figure 5.1).

Beta-blockers

Adrenaline and noradrenaline bind to beta-receptors. (Noradrenaline is the transmitter released by the sympathetic nervous system.) This binding increases heart rate, strengthens the force of the heart's contraction, constricts some blood vessels and stimulates the release of renin from the kidney. In turn, renin converts a relatively inactive precursor into angiotensin I (see Figure 5.1). Beta-blockers (or, more fully, beta-adrenergic receptor blockers) prevent adrenaline and noradrenaline from binding to this receptor.

Howard and Ellerbeck note that injecting beta-blockers within 12 to 24 hours of an MI followed by oral treatment with beta-blockers reduces death during the next week by approximately 13 per cent. Overall, treatment lasting from several months to three years reduced total mortality, non-fatal heart attacks and sudden death by approximately 20 to 30 per cent. Although almost everyone benefits, beta-blockers are especially effective in high-risk people – such as the elderly and those with large infarctions, arrhythmias or left ventricular dysfunction.

Thrombolytic drugs: the clot busters

Rapid treatment with a thrombolytic drug breaks down the blood clot (thrombus) blocking the coronary artery. This restores blood flow to the heart, limiting further damage and encouraging healing. The sooner blood flow is restored (reperfusion), the better your chances of surviving and the less damage your heart endures. So, doctors inject thrombolytic drugs as soon as they're sure you've suffered a heart attack.

Starting streptokinase (a widely used thrombolytic) within 1.5 to 3 hours of a heart attack results in reperfusion in up to 90 per cent of cases. In a trial called GISSI, 13 per cent of those who received a placebo died within 21 days of suffering a heart attack compared to just under 11 per cent of those treated with streptokinase. In the ISIS-2 study, 12 per cent of people with a suspected heart attack who received placebo died from vascular disease within five weeks, compared to 9 per cent of those treated with streptokinase, NICE notes.

NICE recommends starting thrombolysis as soon as possible, normally within 12 hours of the onset of symptoms of a heart attack. As time is of the essence, ambulance paramedics may inject thrombolytic drugs. Administering thrombolytic drugs before reaching hospital reduces deaths by 17 per cent compared to waiting until admission.

Clots, bacteria and heart attacks

In 1933, William Smith Tillett, working at Johns Hopkins University in Baltimore, noted that streptococci, a type of bacteria, clumped in test tubes that contained human plasma – the yellow fluid in which blood cells float – but not in test tubes that contained serum. Unlike plasma, serum doesn't contain proteins responsible for blood clots. So, as Sikri and Bardia recount, a 'factor' in plasma that is absent in serum must cause the clumping. As part of his investigations, Tillett triggered clot formation in five test tubes filled with human plasma, two of which contained streptococci. After several hours, the tubes containing streptococci showed a layer of liquid. Tillett concluded that streptococci released a chemical that dissolved clots. Further tests identified streptokinase as the clot-busting chemical and found it activated plasminogen, a protein produced by the liver. Plasminogen is present in plasma and most tissue fluids – but it's inactive. Chemicals produced by the body, a thrombus, or a thrombolytic drug covert plasminogen into plasmin. In turn, plasmin dissolves blood clots.

Another thrombolytic drug, alteplase, reached clinics in the late 1980s. Alteplase is a genetically engineered version of the protein that naturally activates plasminogen. Doctors and paramedics give other, more recently introduced, thrombolytic drugs (e.g. reteplase and tenecteplase) by injection rather than by an infusion (a 'drip' into the vein).

Side effects of thrombolytic drugs

As you might expect from a drug that breaks down clots, uncontrolled bleeding is the most important side effect with thrombolysis. For example, NICE comments, up to one person in 100 receiving a thrombolytic suffers a haemorrhagic stroke. The risk increases as you get older and if you have raised blood pressure. Thrombolysis can also cause poorly controlled bleeding at injection sites, in the gastrointestinal tract or elsewhere, as well as dangerously low blood pressure (hypotension). So, people with bleeding disorders (e.g. haemophilia) or who have recently haemorrhaged, been seriously injured, undergone surgery or suffered a recent stroke might not be suitable for thrombolysis.

Streptokinase comes from a bacterium (see above). So, your immune system will think it's under attack. Within 2 or 3 days, you'll produce antibodies, which can remain in your system for years. These antibodies may reduce the efficacy of subsequent streptokinase treatment and increase your risk of suffering a severe allergic reaction. So doctors tend to give streptokinase once per patient. If you've had streptokinase before, you (or your carer) should tell the ambulance or A&E team. Doctors should give you a card that you can carry with you.

Heparin

Heparin is one of the oldest drugs still commonly used by doctors. Researchers first isolated heparin in 1916 from liver. (*Hepar* is the Greek for 'liver'.) Rather than breaking clots up, heparin keeps a blood clot from expanding or travelling to another part of your body.

Doctors call the original version of heparin 'unfractionated heparin'. Although unfractionated heparin is often highly effective, the response can fluctuate. So, people taking heparin often need regular, time-consuming monitoring and, in many cases, frequent dose changes. Unfractionated heparin can also cause thrombocytopenia (abnormally low platelet numbers); bleeding complications and osteoporosis (brittle bone disease) during long-term use.

These limitations prompted the development of low molecular weight heparins (LMWHs). The manufacturer uses chemicals or enzymes to break the heparin chain, producing fragments that are around a third of the size. LMWHs produce a more predictable response and require less intensive monitoring. Magee and colleagues found that LMWHs reduced the risk of heart attack in people with acute coronary syndrome by 17 per cent and the need for revascularization procedures by 12 per cent compared with unfractionated heparin. LMWHs may also be less likely to cause bleeding, thrombocytopenia and osteoporosis.

Glycoprotein IIb/IIIa inhibitors

Glycoprotein IIb/IIIa (GP IIb/IIIa) inhibitors (e.g. eptifibatide, tirofiban and abciximab) prevent platelets from aggregating and forming clots. O'Donovan notes that doctors may use GP IIb/IIIa inhibitors to reduce the risk of clots in various circumstances, including:

- people with unstable angina or NSTEMI at intermediate or high risk of further MI or death who are due to undergo angiography in the three days after hospital admission;
- people with unstable angina or NSTEMI who are at high risk of a subsequent heart attack or death;
- alongside heparin or aspirin to prevent clotting before and during elective percutaneous coronary intervention (PCI; see below);
- people with diabetes undergoing elective PCI; and
- people needing complex procedures – such as those requiring several stents (see below).

Percutaneous coronary intervention (PCI)

Apart from drugs, surgeons can unblock clogged coronary arteries. For example, during PCI ('percutaneous' means through the skin), surgeons thread a thin catheter tipped with a balloon and guided by X-ray from an artery in the groin or arm to the blockage in the coronary artery. This technique, introduced in 1977, has several names including percutaneous transluminal coronary angioplasty, coronary artery balloon dilatation or balloon angioplasty. Once the balloon is in place, the surgeon inflates it, which compresses the plaque, widens the artery and improves blood flow.

Doctors call angioplasty that is performed as an emergency treatment for an MI 'primary angioplasty'. However, angioplasty can treat CHD and angina *before* you suffer a heart attack – elective angioplasty – or if you develop angina after coronary artery bypass grafts (CABG; see below). You'll need an angiogram before or at the same time as the angioplasty.

Michaels and Chatterjee comment that balloon angioplasty usually takes 1 to 2 hours. Most people undergoing the procedure only need local anaesthesia and mild sedation. The BHF notes that you'll probably be discharged from hospital two or three days after undergoing angioplasty for a heart attack. The BHF suggests checking the insertion site in your groin or arm when you get home. You'll almost certainly have some bruising. The BHF advises contacting your doctor if you get any redness or swelling or if the bruising worsens. You should discuss with your doctor or nurse what you can do, and when you can do it, after primary or elective angioplasty.

Occasionally, angioplasty completely blocks the coronary artery. As a result, around one in every 1,000 people undergoing angioplasty needs a coronary artery bypass graft (CABG), the BHF comment. In less than one in 100 cases – the risk depends on your health and your heart condition – angioplasty may trigger an MI or stroke. There is also a risk that the area could become blocked again after a seemingly successful operation – re-stenosis. In general, the benefits far outweigh the risks. But if you are considering elective angioplasty (i.e. it's not an emergency), you should talk the risks and benefits over with your cardiologist.

The causes of re-stenosis

According to NICE, re-stenosis arises from three main causes. First, the artery can recoil when the surgeon deflates the balloon. The recoil is usually either immediate or occurs within 24 hours of angioplasty and may require emergency CABG. Stents almost eliminate recoil. Secondly, the tunica adventitia (see Chapter 1) can contract as a response to injury to the vessel caused by the balloon, causing re-stenosis between three and six months after the procedure. Finally, the balloon can trigger an increase in the amount of muscle in the arterial wall, usually between four and six months after the angioplasty, causing the vessel to contract. Around 20 per cent of people undergoing relatively straightforward surgery need revascularization. The risk is higher – up to 50 per cent – in those needing more complicated surgery, those who received a saphenous vein CABG (see below) or those who have diabetes.

Stents

In 1986, surgeons started inserting a wire-mesh tube called a stent to keep the artery open. Initially, they used stents to treat complications during balloon dilation (such as recoil). Stents reduced re-stenosis rates following balloon angioplasty from 30–40 per cent to 20–25 per cent. Today, surgeons implant a stent during around 95 per cent of PCIs to maintain blood flow.

The surgeon slips a 'collapsed' stent over the balloon catheter and moves the tube next to the blockage. When the surgeon inflates the balloon, the stent expands and remains in place after the balloon deflates. The stent improves blood flow to the heart muscle and often relieves symptoms such as chest pain. Within a few weeks of stent placement, the artery's inside lining covers the metal scaffold. This covering allows blood to flow easily over the stent without clotting, Dangas and Kuepper note. However, scar tissue forms underneath the healthy lining. In around a quarter of cases, thick scar tissue can obstruct blood flow – called in-stent re-stenosis.

Typically, in-stent re-stenosis emerges three to six months after the procedure. In-stent re-stenosis is unlikely to emerge more than 12 months after the stent was implanted. Dangas and Kuepper note that the symptoms arising from in-stent re-stenosis are similar to those that initially prompted the implantation – such as chest pain triggered by exercise. People with diabetes, however, may have fewer or unusual symptoms. Fortunately, however, in-stent re-stenosis rarely leads to heart attacks.

Because of the risk of in-stent re-stenosis, doctors increasingly use drug-eluting stents, which reduce re-stenosis rates by between 60 and 80 per cent. (Stents that don't release drugs are called bare metal stents.) Re-stenosis occurs when cells in the blood vessel wall divide, triggered in part by inflammation. So, some stents release paclitaxel, which inhibits cell division. Other drug-eluting stents release sirolimus or everolimus, which reduce inflammation. The concentration of these drugs is high around the stent. But very little reaches the rest of the body, reducing the risk of side effects elsewhere.

Brachytherapy

Doctors can treat in-stent re-stenosis using intracoronary radiotherapy (brachytherapy). The surgeon uses balloon angioplasty to open the blocked vessels and leaves a catheter that releases a small amount of radiation in the vessel for several minutes. The irradiated tissue is less likely to grow within the stent, reducing the risk of another re-stenosis.

People receiving a stent usually take aspirin and an antiplatelet drug (such as clopidogrel, ticagrelor or prasugrel) to reduce the risk of clotting. As aspirin and antiplatelet drugs act through different mechanisms, the combination is more effective than either alone. Vlaar and colleagues concluded that clopidogrel increased the likelihood of rapid reperfusion by 51 per cent, while reducing deaths by 53 per cent and the risk of death or another MI by 46 per cent compared to aspirin alone. (People in the study also received heparin.) However, clopidogrel produces a more variable platelet response and has a slower onset of action than ticagrelor or prasugrel. As these drugs block blood clotting, you could experience uncontrolled bleeds. Some people experience breathlessness with ticagrelor. Your doctor will help you decide the best combination for you.

Coronary artery bypass graft (CABG)

CABG tends to be used when atherosclerosis causes severe narrowing or blockage of the left main coronary artery or affects at least two coronary arteries. However, surgeons may be unable to operate on very small coronary arteries, Michaels and Chatterjee point out. A double bypass refers to two grafts, a triple bypass to three grafts, quadruple to four and so on. Obviously, a quintuple bypass is much more serious than receiving a single graft.

During CABG, the surgeon removes a section of healthy blood vessel from the leg (saphenous vein), the chest (internal mammary artery) or the arm (radial artery). The surgeon uses this 'graft' to create a detour or bypass around the blocked coronary artery. A heart–lung machine maintains the blood's circulation during the operation. Doctors may use GP IIb/IIIa inhibitors to prevent blood clotting during the operation. You will need general anaesthesia, will probably spend several days in hospital and may take several months to recover fully.

The choice of angioplasty or CABG depends on the potential risks and benefits in your case. In other words, the balance is different for an otherwise healthy person with a single blocked vessel from the risk and benefits in someone with diabetes or heart failure and four narrow arteries. If you're planning to have the operation, discuss the risks fully with your cardiologist.

Keyhole CABG

Keyhole surgery may make CABG less traumatic. Michaels and Chatterjee note that a relatively new technique called minimally invasive direct coronary artery bypass (MIDCAB) does not require a heart–lung machine – the surgeon performs the operation on a 'stabilized' but still beating heart. Rather than cutting through the breastbone (sternum), the surgeon operates through a small incision between the ribs. MIDCAB is less traumatic with less scarring (2–3 inches compared to 6–8 inches), involves a shorter hospital stay and usually means the recovery is more rapid than with conventional CABG. However, MIDCAB is generally suitable for by-passing only one or two blocked arteries.

Defibrillation

A heart attack can cause a marked disturbance in the heart's rhythm – an arrhythmia. In some cases, the heart may beat hundreds of times a minute. Ventricular fibrillation is the deadliest arrhythmia. During ventricular fibrillation, the heart's electrical activity is chaotic. So, the ventricles stop pumping and quiver uncontrollably ('fibrillate'), causing a cardiac arrest (see page 13). Doctors or paramedics may give a large electric shock, using a defibrillator, which often restores the normal heartbeat. But they need to act quickly. According to the BHF, the chances of surviving a cardiac arrest decline by 14 per cent for each minute that passes without restarting the heart.

So, automatic external defibrillators, which diagnose the problem and deliver the appropriate pulse of electricity, are available increasingly in planes, at workplaces, in homes and in other locations.

If an automated defibrillator isn't available, you should call 999 immediately and start cardiopulmonary resuscitation – mouth-to-mouth resuscitation and chest compression to keep the blood moving – until the ambulance arrives. (Emergency ambulances carry defibrillators.) Paramedics may inject a person in cardiac arrest with adrenaline. Jacobs and colleagues remark that adrenaline 'restarts' the heart three times more often than placebo (24 per cent and 8 per cent of cases, respectively).

Remember that unless defibrillation or cardiopulmonary resuscitation starts within three to four minutes, the BHF warns that the person may suffer permanent brain damage. If you're the partner or carer of someone with heart disease it's especially important to learn cardiopulmonary resuscitation. You could contact the St John Ambulance or the British Red Cross for details of first aid courses in your area.

6

After a heart attack

A heart attack is usually a sign that you have atherosclerosis. But once you've recovered, the underlying disease could still be lurking in your blood vessels. So, once you've suffered one heart attack, you're at increased risk of suffering another. Haffner and colleagues noted that a fifth of heart attack survivors suffer another MI in the next seven years. Almost half of those with diabetes will have another heart attack. This means that treatment to help you survive an MI doesn't end when you're discharged from hospital. Secondary prevention is vital to ensure your long-term survival. That means taking your medicines regularly as prescribed by your doctor and making lifestyle changes (see Chapter 7). Modern medicines, despite their efficacy, do not replace a healthy lifestyle. But they're an invaluable safety net.

After your discharge, you'll probably receive one or more medicines. The choice depends on your particular problems – for example, whether you develop heart failure and whether there are medical reasons why you can't take certain drugs. For instance, you may receive angiotensin receptor blockers if you can't take ACE inhibitors. The following are examples:

- Aspirin to help prevent further heart attacks by reducing the risk of blood clots. You may take clopidogrel (see page 69) if you can't take aspirin. You may receive warfarin if you can take neither aspirin nor clopidogrel.
- Diuretics, ACE inhibitors or angiotensin receptor blockers (see Chapter 5), which reduce blood pressure, alleviate breathlessness and treat heart failure.
- Nitrates, calcium channel blockers or beta-blockers, which alleviate angina by reducing the amount of oxygen the heart requires or increasing blood flow through coronary arteries, or both. Beta-blockers also reduce the risk of death after an MI.
- Drugs to control risk factors such as high cholesterol levels or

dangerously raised blood pressure (hypertension) – we shall look at these problems in Chapter 7.

- Anti-arrhythmic drugs (see page 77) to ensure the rhythm of your heart is normal.

Despite these drugs and despite the best efforts of the medical team, the patient and the family, several problems can follow in the wake of a heart attack. So, this chapter also looks at some complications as well as the good news, such as when you can return to work and to driving.

How diuretics work

Your kidneys filter water, salts and some waste products from your blood. Healthy kidneys reabsorb most of the water and essential salts, such as sodium. But some remains with the waste products, forming urine. Diuretics ('water tablets') reduce the amount of sodium and water that is reabsorbed. In response, you produce more urine. So, the volume and, therefore, pressure of blood falls. In turn, your heart doesn't have to work as hard.

Calcium channel blockers

Most of the calcium in your body (about 1 kg in a 70 kg person) helps build strong bones and teeth. Around 1 per cent has other critical roles, such as ensuring efficient transmission of signals along nerves, controlling hormone secretion and allowing muscle contraction. For example, calcium allows the myocardium and the rings of muscle that control the diameter of blood vessels (which help maintain blood pressure) to contract properly.

Calcium needs to be inside cells to work. So calcium moves through proteins that form 'tunnels' through the membrane that surrounds each cell. Changes in the shape of this 'channel' control the flow of calcium by opening or closing the pore that runs through the centre. This allows calcium into the cell – rather like raising or lowering the barrier that controls the flow of road traffic through a tunnel.

Calcium channel blockers (calcium antagonists) inhibit the influx of calcium through these tunnels. The decline in calcium inside the muscle cell dilates blood vessels and so lowers blood pressure. Some calcium channel blockers also reduce the force and rate at which the heart contracts.

Heart failure

Each year, around 27,000 people learn that they've developed heart failure, caused when the heart 'fails' to pump enough blood to meet your organs' demands. Doctors divide heart failure into left and right forms. Eventually, most people with heart failure develop both to a greater or lesser extent.

- In left heart failure (left ventricular systolic dysfunction), the left ventricle cannot pump enough of the blood that it receives from the lungs. Blood backs up in the lungs (pulmonary oedema), causing breathlessness. This is potentially fatal.
- In right heart failure, the right ventricle cannot pump enough of the blood received from the body. So, blood backs up in the legs, ankles, torso and so on, causing peripheral oedema (congestion – which is why doctors refer to congestive heart failure). While peripheral oedema isn't immediately life-threatening, the fluid usually causes discomfort and may produce skin ulcers.

Cardiac asthma

Pulmonary oedema reduces oxygen transfer across the alveoli, causing symptoms – including shortness of breath, coughing and wheezing – that are similar to asthma. So distinguishing the two conditions sometimes proves difficult. Furthermore, asthma and congestive heart failure both commonly cause symptoms during the night. But congestive heart failure generally causes symptoms between one and two hours after lying down, rather than in the early morning as is typical of asthma. Furthermore, ankle swelling and weight gain are unusual in asthma. However, asthma and heart disease are both common. So some people develop both conditions. Treating heart failure reduces pulmonary oedema and, therefore, alleviates cardiac asthma. But some asthma treatments, such as bronchodilators, can exacerbate heart failure and may provoke arrhythmias. My book *Coping with Adult Asthma* offers further advice.

Atherosclerosis in coronary arteries and scars from MIs, which can prevent the heart from beating properly, may lead to heart failure. Heart failure can also arise from other causes, including excessive alcohol consumption (see page 101), hypertension, congenital heart defects, infection of the heart valves (endocarditis) or heart muscle (myocarditis), and left ventricular hypertrophy (LVH).

LVH describes the enlargement (hypertrophy) of the left ventricle caused when a disease or lifestyle factor makes your heart work excessively hard for a long time. As the workload increases, the ventricle thickens, becomes less elastic and eventually fails to pump with as much force as a healthy heart. Hypertension is the most common cause of LVH. The left ventricle works harder to counter raised blood pressure. LVH can also follow, for example:

- aortic valve stenosis (narrowing of the valve separating the left ventricle from the aorta);
- intense, prolonged endurance and strength training;
- obesity.

LVH usually develops gradually and you may not suffer symptoms, especially during the early stages. As LVH progresses, you may experience shortness of breath, chest pain, palpitations, dizziness and fainting, and you may quickly feel exhausted with physical activity. See your doctor if you experience any of these symptoms. The enlarged muscle may also compresses coronary arteries, restricting the heart's blood supply. As a result, you may develop heart failure, arrhythmias, angina, cardiac arrest and heart attacks.

There's not space to discuss treatment for heart failure – it's almost a book in its own right. (Contact your doctor, nurse or the BHF for more details.) However, NICE suggests that people who have heart failure and left ventricular systolic dysfunction after a heart attack should start using a type of diuretic called an aldosterone antagonist within 3–14 days of the MI, preferably after beginning an ACE inhibitor.

Atrial fibrillation and other arrhythmias

Arrhythmias are changes in the heart's rate or rhythm. The heart may beat too quickly (tachycardia), too slowly (bradycardia) or irregularly. Most arrhythmias are harmless, but some are serious or even life-threatening. For example, ventricular arrhythmias may cause cardiac arrest. So, always check with your GP if you suffer regular or persistent palpitations.

Atrial fibrillation (AF) – uncontrolled quivering of the upper chambers of the heart (the atria) – is common after a MI and dramatically undermines your survival chances. For example:

- Crenshaw and colleagues found that around 10 per cent of people who have had a heart attack show AF either when they reach hospital or during the 30 days after their MI. AF almost trebled the risk of stroke while in hospital compared to people without arrhythmia (around 3 per cent and 1 per cent, respectively). People with AF were more than twice as likely to be dead after 30 days (14 per cent and 6 per cent, respectively) and after a year (22 per cent and 9 per cent, respectively).
- Stewart and collaborators reported that 89 per cent of women and 66 per cent of men with AF died or were hospitalized with cardiovascular events over 20 years. This compared to 27 per cent of women and 45 per cent of men without AF. And AF doubled to trebled the risk of cardiovascular events, fatal or non-fatal strokes and heart failure, and roughly doubled deaths from any cause.
- Jabre and colleagues reported that 9 per cent of people who had had a heart attack showed AF before admission. Another 23 per cent developed AF after their MI. During an average of just over six-and-a-half years, AF increased mortality almost four-fold.

In AF, the atria beat up to 400 times per minute. So, they only partly contract. And a relatively small proportion of the impulses reaches the ventricles. As a result, atrial and ventricular contractions are uncoordinated. In AF, the ventricles usually contract between 140 and 180 times a minute and the force of the contractions varies considerably. Because the heart pumps less effectively, people with AF experience breathlessness (often the first symptom), palpitations and dizziness.

Initially, a person usually experiences isolated attacks of AF. Over time, however, the attacks often become increasingly persistent, and eventually may cause potentially serious complications. For example, AF may underlie up to a quarter of strokes. Indeed, AF increases the risk of stroke between four- and five-fold, Benjamin and colleagues note, doubles the risk of dementia and triples the risk of heart failure. So, ask your doctor or nurse to measure your pulse. Everyone who has an irregular pulse should have an ECG whether or not they experience symptoms.

Pacemakers

A pacemaker is a small, battery-operated device usually implanted under the skin of your chest. When sensors detect abnormal heart rhythm, the pacemaker sends electrical pulses to trigger a normal heartbeat. According to the NHS, surgeons implant about 25,000 pacemakers every year in the UK to treat heart block (irregular or slow heartbeats because the electrical signals are not transmitted properly), bradycardia and heart failure.

Treating arrhythmias

Mild arrhythmias often don't need treatment. Your doctor may recommend surgery or drugs (antiarrhythmics) if your arrhythmia causes serious symptoms (such as dizziness, chest pain or fainting) or if you're at increased risk of heart failure, stroke or cardiac arrest.

Doctors may treat AF with beta-blockers, calcium channel blockers and digoxin (digitalis) to slow the racing heart. During AF, the heart does not pump blood completely out of the chambers. So, blood may pool and clot. Some clots may travel from the heart and block an artery, causing a stroke or heart attack. So some people with certain arrhythmias (including AF) also receive medicines (such as warfarin, dabigatran, heparin, rivaroxaban and aspirin) that reduce the risk of blood clots. Surgeons can also tackle arrhythmias in several other ways. For example:

- Pacemakers accelerate dangerously slow heart rate.
- A jolt of electricity (cardioversion or defibrillation) can establish normal heart rate.
- In people at high risk of life-threatening ventricular fibrillation, surgeons may insert an implantable cardioverter defibrillator (ICD) under the skin in the chest.
- Perform CABG to treat arrhythmias arising from CHD.
- Destroy small areas of heart tissue that generate the arrhythmia (cardiac ablation).

There's not space to examine the pros and cons of each of these methods here. It's worth discussing the most appropriate treatment with your cardiologist and check out the information from the BHF and other patient groups.

Stable angina

Almost 2.1 million people in the UK endure the crippling pain of angina. Overall, around one in 20 men and one in 25 women suffer from angina, the BHF estimates. However, the risk rises sharply with advancing age: just under a quarter of men and one in six women aged more than 75 years suffer angina. And every year, UK doctors diagnose 28,000 new cases.

When the heart works harder – during exercise or at times of heightened emotion, for example – narrowed coronary arteries mean that the heart's demand for oxygen can exceed supply. This imbalance causes chest pain or discomfort. Nitroglycerin (glyceryl trinitrate or GTN) opens the vessels supplying the heart, so alleviating the pain. You place the GTN tablet, or spray the medicine, under your tongue (sublingually) to get the drug into your blood stream rapidly. Rest also restores the balance and so alleviates the pain. However, some arteries narrowed by more than 70 per cent can trigger angina at rest.

Apart from, or as well as, atherosclerosis, several other conditions can trigger angina. For example, some people suffer an attack at night (nocturnal angina) – in part because of the natural cardiovascular rhythms (see page 20). Lying down may trigger angina because gravity redistributes the body's fluids, which makes the heart work harder (angina decubitus). Several cardiovascular diseases can cause angina, including: severe hypertension; abnormal, narrow or leaking aortic valves; and thickening of the walls of the heart chambers (cardiomyopathy).

Angina symptoms vary markedly. Most people with angina report heaviness, tightness, pressure or pain in the centre of the chest or beneath the breastbone that generally lasts between 2 and 15 minutes. (As we've seen, the pain of a heart attack typically lasts longer than this.) The pain, which can be severe, may spread from the chest to the left shoulder and arm to the neck or left jaw, throat, teeth, back or stomach. Some people may feel nauseous or breathless, or both.

Try to indentify your angina triggers. You could keep a diary of when your symptoms emerged, how you felt and what you were doing when the attack developed. Apart from exercise and emotions, large meals, rapid changes in temperature, sleep deprivation and severe anaemia can trigger angina. So it might be worth asking your doctor to check, especially if you're a vegetarian (meat is the best natural source of iron) or lose a lot of blood due to heavy menstrual periods.

Keeping a diary can also help you identify ways to self-manage angina, such as pacing your activities and setting goals. Your cardiac rehabilitation team (see page 85) or GP can help, such as advising about safe levels of physical exertion, including sex. You should also discuss ways to manage stress, anxiety or depression. As we've seen, strong emotions commonly trigger angina. As mentioned before, you should tell your GP or cardiac team as soon as the pattern of your angina changes. The angina diary will aid your discussion.

Drugs for angina

Your doctor will probably prescribe a short-acting nitrate, usually sublingual GTN, for your angina. Apart from alleviating the attack, you should use the short-acting nitrate immediately before any planned exercise or exertion. However, because nitrates dilate blood vessels, they can cause flushing, headache and light-headedness. If you suffer light-headedness, sit down or find something to hold on to. If the pain doesn't disappear after 5 minutes, NICE suggests taking a second dose. You should call 999 if the pain isn't gone 5 minutes after the second dose.

In addition, your doctor will probably suggest you take either a beta-blocker or a calcium channel blocker to prevent angina attacks. If the beta-blocker does not control angina adequately or you develop side effects, you can switch to the calcium channel blocker, or vice versa. Some people need both a beta-blocker and a calcium channel blocker. In some cases – such as if side effects remain a problem – NICE suggests trying one of the following medicines: a long-acting nitrate; ivabradine; nicorandil; or ranolazine. If these fail to control your angina, your doctor may suggest CABG or PCI.

Other complications of an MI

Several other complications, such as pericarditis, can follow in the wake of an MI. In pericarditis, the heart attack inflames the pericardium, the thin sac-like membrane covering the heart's outer surface. The pericardium helps stop the heart from moving in the chest when you're active.

In other cases, a heart weakened by an MI, arrhythmia or one of several other cardiac conditions suddenly cannot pump enough blood to meet the body's needs. This is called cardiogenic shock and is a much more profound reduction in oxygen supply than occurs in heart failure. Indeed, it's fatal unless treated immediately. About one in 14 people who suffer a heart attack develops cardiogenic shock, which is a leading cause of death among people in hospital after an MI.

Prompt treatment to restore cardiac blood flow and help the heart pump more efficiently means that around half of the people who go into cardiogenic shock now survive. The fall in oxygen supply causes the symptoms of shock (Table 6.1), which can also arise from several other causes. Whatever the cause, if you think someone is in shock, you should call 999 or for medical assistance in hospital immediately.

Table 6.1 Symptoms of shock

Confusion or lack of alertness
Loss of consciousness
Sudden and persistently rapid heartbeat
Weak pulse
Sweating
Pale skin
Rapid breathing
Reduced (or no) urine output
Cool hands and feet

A heart attack can also kill cells in – and punch holes through – the wall separating the ventricles (septal rupture). The damage means that the ventricles can't pump efficiently, and ventricular septal rupture can precipitate cardiogenic shock. MIs can also damage the papillary muscles, which anchor the bicuspid (mitral) and tricuspid valves (see Chapter 1). So, blood doesn't flow correctly between the heart's chambers. Again, this can trigger cardiogenic shock.

Depression and other psychiatric problems

Depression is more than feeling 'down in the dumps'. It's profound, debilitating mental and physical lethargy, a pervasive sense of worthlessness and intense, deep, unshakable sadness. If you've never experienced depression, it's difficult to appreciate how devastating the condition is. Unfortunately, depression is common after heart attacks and unstable angina, and undermines survival. For example, Lespérance and colleagues found that two-fifths of those hospitalized with unstable angina were clinically depressed. Depressed people were almost seven times more likely to die from cardiac causes or suffer a non-fatal heart attack during the next year than those who were not depressed. Furthermore, Frasure-Smith and co-authors reported that depression increased the risk of death over the six months after a heart attack around four-fold.

Suffering a heart attack or unstable angina can cause other psychiatric conditions. For example, Pedersen and colleagues note that around a quarter of people who suffer acute coronary syndrome develop post-traumatic stress disorder (PTSD). Fear of death during the attack seems to increase the chance of PTSD.

The link between the mind and the heart runs both ways. Psychiatric disorders can trigger heart attacks, as INTERHEART showed (see page 26). Furthermore, deaths from cardiovascular disease, lethal arrhythmias and heart attacks rise immediately after intensely stressful disasters such as earthquakes and terrorist attacks, O'Keefe and colleagues remark. Negative emotions, depression and the type D personality also seem to increase the risk of developing and dying from heart disease.

The type D personality and heart attack

People with type D personalities (the D stands for 'distressed') experience persistent negative emotions, pessimism and social inhibition (such as being intensely shy and introspective). So, while people with type D personalities are especially anxious, irritable and depressed, fear of disapproval means that they don't share these emotions. Denollet and collaborators noted that people with type D personalities were three times more likely to need angioplasty or CABG, or to suffer from cardiovascular problems such as heart failure, heart transplantation, MI, peripheral artery disease and death. Counsellors and psychotherapists may be able to help you develop better coping strategies.

Indeed, even just feeling 'unsatisfied' with your life can increase your risk of heart disease. Compared to British civil servants reporting low levels of life satisfaction, those who said they were moderately and highly satisfied were 20 per cent and 26 per cent less likely to develop CHD, respectively, allowing for other risk factors. Satisfaction with their job, family life, sex life and themselves each reduced CHD risk by around 12 per cent, Boehm and colleagues report.

A reduced risk of angina seemed to account for much of the reduced CHD risk seen in this study. Compared to civil servants reporting low levels of life satisfaction, those who said they were moderately and highly satisfied were 24 per cent and 41 per cent less likely to experience angina, respectively.

Boehm and colleagues report that considered individually, marital and love relationships, leisure and standard of living did not influence CHD risk. However, as we'll see in Chapter 8, a supportive relationship can improve the long-term chances of surviving a heart attack. Indeed, social connections, optimism, humour, altruism, animal companionship and involvement in organized religion seem to protect against cardiovascular disease.

Get treatment

So, it's important to get help for depression, anxiety or any other psychiatric conditions, whether these emerge before or after your heart attack. If symptoms markedly affect your daily life, the doctor may suggest anti-depressants or drugs to alleviate anxiety. Don't dismiss drugs out of hand. It's often difficult to plan the best way of reducing your risk of heart disease in particular or of tackling your life problems in general when you're carrying the burden imposed by depression or anxiety. While drugs can ease the symptoms, they don't cure the problem. Nevertheless, medicines may offer you a 'window of opportunity' to improve your control of your heart disease and deal with any other issues you face.

'Talking therapies' may also help. Your GP may be able to recommend a local counsellor, who can help patients and their partners identify and manage the practical, psychological and emotional challenges that arise when living with a chronic condition, such as heart disease. Alternatively, you could contact the British Association for Counselling and Psychotherapy. It might be worth trying to find a counsellor or therapist who has experience helping people with heart disease. Some people also find that complementary therapies help them relax and tackle the stress of living with a chronic disease (see page 108).

Returning to work

Returning to work helps reduce the risk of depression – partly because it's a sign your life is getting back to normal. According to the BHF, around a third of people who suffer a heart attack in the UK are under 65 years of age. Two-thirds of these are in employment when they suffer their MI, but up to half never return to work. Many probably could have worked, although they may need several months to recover.

MIs usually take at least five to six weeks to heal. So, people usually return to work after a doctor has reviewed the survivor's health at least two months after the heart attack. You and your cardiac team need to strike a delicate balance. The longer you wait the less likely you are to return to work. But you don't want to trigger another heart attack. So, if tests show only minimal heart damage you may be able to return to work sooner – talk it over with your cardiologist. On the other hand, the BHF notes that most people who have survived a cardiac arrest or undergone CABG take longer to recover physically and mentally, and may need up to six months off work.

Nevertheless, some people return to work after a severe heart attack, while others remain off work after a relatively minor MI. Several factors influence your chances of returning to work. Persistent symptoms – such as angina and breathlessness – may reduce the chance of returning to work or at least delay your return. Depressed people, not surprisingly, are less likely than those with a more optimistic outlook to return to work after a MI. However, your health beliefs are arguably the most influential factor. For example, the BHF notes that people who believe that stress at work caused their heart attack will probably be reluctant to return. Other people believe that their heart is 'worn out' and they need to 'take things easy' – which means giving up their job. And people who believe that their heart attack will have a long-term impact on their health are much less likely to return to work than those who see the MI as a 'short-term' problem.

On the other hand, doctors and employers are more likely to 'allow' a person to go back to a sedentary job (and especially to return quickly) than to a job that involves manual labour. However, the BHF notes that little scientific evidence supports this caution. Very few jobs ban a return to work following a heart attack – deep sea diving being one. Even some professional civil pilots may resume flying if they pass a stringent medical examination after being grounded for several months.

People who work in jobs demanding 'heavy manual labour' can usually return following the 'all-clear' from a cardiologist, which may involve an exercise test. Nevertheless, people with heart problems should not lift and carry objects that are so heavy that they need to hold their breath. But lifting such weights isn't a good idea for anyone other than strength athletes – the risk of injuring muscle, tendons, ligaments and so on is considerable.

Against this background, your cardiac rehabilitation programme (see below) should include advice about whether and when you can return to work. Occasionally, the therapist may need to assess the work place. If your heart attack reduced your exercise tolerance or the work is physically demanding, your cardiology team may suggest a programme of 'work-hardening'. You and the team should work together to develop a plan that minimizes the impact of fatigue, poor concentration and other symptoms that can follow in the wake of an MI. For example, the BHF suggests beginning with half-days at work and light or less challenging duties, rather than throwing yourself immediately back into the fray, and gradually building up over two to three weeks. You may need additional rest periods if fatigue is a problem or your return to work is delayed – such as after CABG.

Driving

Most drivers don't need to inform the Driver and Vehicle Licensing Authority (DVLA) that they've suffered a heart attack or angina or undergone CABG. Generally, if you make an uncomplicated recovery from a heart attack or CABG you can start driving after at least a month. You must stop driving for at least one week after successful angioplasty. If the PCI wasn't successful, you should stop driving for at least four weeks. However, even if the time's up, you should make sure you're confident that you could control the vehicle – such as being able to perform an emergency stop without discomfort – before getting back behind the wheel. And always wait until your doctor tells you that you are fit to restart driving. If you are in doubt call the DVLA or your doctor.

According to the DVLA you may continue to drive if you have angina unless you suffer attacks at rest, while driving or with emotion. If so, you should stop driving until your symptoms are under control. If you suffer an angina attack while driving, you should pull over, rest and take your angina medication. Once your symptoms resolve, you can restart your journey. If you can, it might be worth switching drivers. And try to avoid road rage: stress can trigger angina.

You must cease driving and tell the DVLA if you have a heart condition that may cause sudden attacks of disabling giddiness or fainting, which may be the case if a surgeon has implanted a pacemaker or a cardioverter defibrillator. Speak to your cardiologist, GP or rehabilitation nurse if you're unsure. If you hold a large goods vehicle or passenger-carrying vehicle licence you must inform the DVLA if you suffer a heart attack. You may be able to keep your licence after a medical assessment in all these cases. The DVLA issues regular updates on driving restrictions (<www.direct.gov.uk/driverhealth>). You will need to let your insurance companies (for driving, life and any other policies) know that you have suffered a heart attack.

Cardiac rehabilitation programmes

Most MI survivors join a cardiac rehabilitation programme, usually starting four to eight weeks after the heart attack. People who have undergone or are waiting for CABG, revascularization or other heart operations, or who suffer from heart failure or angina, may also join. The members of the cardiac rehabilitation team will depend on your needs, but may include a cardiologist, specialist cardiac nurse, physiotherapist, exercise specialist, occupational therapist, dietician and psychologist. It's also worth making an appointment to see your GP once you're discharged from hospital.

Typically, the programme includes lifestyle advice and advice on how to manage stress, anxiety and depression, as well as a considerable emphasis on exercise. According to the NHS, exercise programmes for cardiac rehabilitation reduce all-cause and cardiovascular mortality by about 25 per cent among heart attack survivors. Even programmes without exercise reduce all-cause mortality by around 13 per cent. The programme will help you set goals and advise on when you can return to work, start to drive again and resume your sex life. They'll also help you understand the risks and benefits of treatment.

In many cases, you'll go once or twice a week for about six to eight weeks. It's worth making the effort. The cardiac rehabilitation programme helps rebuild your confidence and you'll meet other people who can offer mutual support. If you've not been invited to a cardiac rehabilitation programme, ask at your hospital or GP surgery. However, while the rehabilitation programme lasts a few months, changes in exercise, diet and smoking cessation should last the rest of your life – as we'll see in Chapter 7.

7

Preventing another heart attack

Your chances of surviving a heart attack are better than ever. About half of people now survive even cardiogenic shock, a complication that until relatively recently almost always proved fatal. But, as we've seen, having one heart attack means you're much more likely to suffer another. Remember than a heart attack is a symptom and not the disease. So, to survive long term you should take your medicines and follow a heart-healthy lifestyle to tackle the underlying atherosclerosis.

Assessing risk

As we saw in Chapter 2, heart attack risk factors are often synergistic and usually cluster. So, doctors use charts that consider important factors – diabetes, hypertension, smoking and so on – and set a 'threshold' for 'unacceptable' risk. So, doctors may consider a 20 per cent or more risk of developing cardiovascular disease over the next 10 years as unacceptable. They'll tailor your treatment based on your risk.

However, risk is in the eye of the beholder. Personally, I'd regard a 10 per cent risk of developing cardiovascular disease over the next 10 years as unacceptable. But your doctor may not actively treat this level of risk. Drugs cause side effects and they may regard the dangers as outweighing the benefits. Nevertheless, you can still change your lifestyle to reduce your heart attack risk. For example, INTERHEART identified four factors that reduce your risk of suffering a heart attack:

- Not smoking reduced the risk of suffering the first MI by 65 per cent.
- Eating fruit and vegetables daily reduced MI risk by 30 per cent.
- Moderate exercise (walking, cycling or gardening) or strenuous

exercise (jogging, football and vigorous swimming) for at least four hours a week cut the risk by 14 per cent.

- Regular alcohol consumption (three or more times a week) reduced MI risk by 9 per cent.

And the healthier your lifestyle the lower the risk:

- Not smoking and eating fruit and vegetables daily reduced MI risk by 76 per cent.
- Not smoking, eating fruit and vegetables daily and regular exercise cut MI risk by 79 per cent.
- Not smoking, eating fruit and vegetables daily, regular exercise and regular alcohol consumption cut MI risk by 81 per cent.

INTERHEART looked at the risk of the first heart attack. But the same principles apply to further heart attacks after your first MI, as we'll see in this chapter. Indeed, because you're at higher risk, the benefits of tackling the factors could be even greater if you've already had a heart attack. In this chapter, we'll look at some ways you and your doctor can help reduce your risk of suffering another heart attack. Remember that drugs do not replace lifestyle changes. You'll need to take the drugs regularly *and* adopt a healthier lifestyle to have the best chance of surviving long-term.

Quit smoking

Nicotine, the addictive chemical in tobacco, and the plant's scientific name (*Nicotiana tabacum*) 'honour' Jean Nicot de Villemain (1530–1600), the French ambassador to Portugal, who introduced tobacco to Parisian society when he returned from Lisbon in 1561. Ironically, the Portuguese regarded tobacco as a medicine. Tobacco rapidly became fashionable. Today, smoking is increasingly socially unacceptable – just look at the huddles of smokers outside offices, pubs and restaurants. During the 1940s, around 70 per cent of men and 40 per cent of women smoked. According to government statistics, in 2009, 22 per cent of men and 20 per cent of women smoked – about 8.8 million people in England.

Around half of those who don't quit smoking die prematurely from their addiction. Indeed, during 2008 more than 80,000 people died prematurely in England from smoking-related diseases. For example:

- Smokers are roughly twice as likely to die from cancer as non-smokers.
- Smoking increases the likelihood of suffering a stroke up to three-fold.
- Smoking underlies a fifth of deaths among middle-aged people.
- Smoking causes around half of all cases of heart disease.

Women's hearts are at especially high risk, possibly because they extract higher levels of toxins from smoke. Huxley and Woodward found that women are 25 per cent more likely than men to develop CHD as a result of cigarette smoking, after other risk factors have been allowed for.

On the other hand, quitting smoking reduces your likelihood of developing most smoking-related diseases. According to the Department of Health, a lifelong smoker dies, on average, around 10 years sooner than he or she otherwise would. A person who stops smoking at 30 or 40 years of age gains, on average, ten years and nine years of life, respectively. Even a 60-year-old person gains, on average, three years of life by quitting. The risk of heart disease drops markedly in the first 12–18 months after cessation. Three to five years after quitting, cardiovascular risk is no different from that of a non-smoker. O'Keefe and colleagues remark that the risk of death falls by just over a third in people with CHD who quit compared with those who continued smoking.

If the benefits to your health are not enough to make you quit, think of the harm you're doing to your loved ones. Second-hand smoke contains more than 4,000 chemicals, including over 50 carcinogens (cancer-causing chemicals). This chemical cocktail increases the risk of serious diseases – including lung cancer, heart disease, asthma and sudden infant death syndrome – in people who inhale second-hand smoke. For example, the risks that a woman who has never smoked will develop lung cancer and heart disease are 24 per cent and 30 per cent greater, respectively, if she lives with a smoker.

However, fewer than one in every 30 smokers manages to quit annually, and more than half of these relapse within a year. And you need to quit, not cut down. People who reduce cigarette consumption usually inhale more deeply to get the same amount of nicotine. Nevertheless, cutting back seems to increase the likelihood that you'll eventually quit by, in some studies, 70 per cent compared with those who never cut back. In other words, reduction can take you a large step towards kicking the habit. But don't stop there.

You'll need to deal with nicotine's withdrawal symptoms, which can leave you irritable, restless and anxious as well as experiencing insomnia and craving a cigarette. (That's why it's a good idea to ask your family and friends for support – see Chapter 8.) In general, these withdrawal symptoms abate over two weeks or so.

Nicotine replacement therapy (NRT) can alleviate the withdrawal symptoms, making quitting easier. Government statistics suggest that nearly a fifth of smokers buy NRT, which increases quit rates by between 50 and 100 per cent. You can chose from various types of NRT. Patches reduce withdrawal symptoms but have a relatively slow onset of action. Nicotine chewing gum, lozenges, inhalers and nasal spray act more quickly. Talk to your pharmacist or GP to find the right combination for you. If you still find quitting tough even after trying NRT, doctors can prescribe other treatments. But there's no quick fix. You'll still need to be committed to quitting.

Tips to help you quit

Breaking tobacco's hold is tough. On some measures, nicotine is more addictive than heroin and cocaine. But, in addition to using NRT, a few simple hints may make life easier:

- Set a quit date, when you will stop completely. Plan ahead: keep a diary of problems and situations that tempt you to light up, such as coffee, meals, pubs or work breaks.
- Try to find something to take your mind off smoking. If you find yourself smoking when you get home in the evening, try a new hobby or exercise. Most people find that the craving for a cigarette usually only lasts a couple of minutes. Some people find that just sucking a hard sweet helps take their mind off the craving.
- Smoking is expensive. Keep a note of how much you save and spend at least some of it on something for yourself.
- Learn to deal with stress and hunger pangs. Military commanders

from the Thirty Years War to the Second World War encouraged smoking to blunt fear and hunger. Some people find that they become more hungry when they stop smoking, so try to avoid reaching for the chocolate. Have a healthy snack handy. You could try relaxation therapies (page 108) to deal with stress.

- Call the NHS smoking helpline for further support on 0800 169 0169.

Coping with relapses

Nicotine is incredibly addictive and, not surprisingly, many people don't manage to quit first time. But if you relapse, try not to become too dispirited. Regard it as a temporary setback, set another quit date and try again. It's also worth trying to identify why you relapsed. Were you stressed out? If so, why? Was smoking linked to a particular time, place or event? Once you know why you slipped you can develop strategies to stop the problem in the future.

Reducing blood pressure

Hypertension is an important risk factor for heart attacks and strokes. So you'll need to control your blood pressure. In most people, 'realistic changes in diet and lifestyle' reduce diastolic blood pressure by 2–3 mmHg, Law and colleagues comment. But some

Table 7.1 Lifestyle changes' impact on blood pressure

Lifestyle change	Reduction in systolic blood pressure
Maintain BMI between 20 and 25 kg/m²	5–10 mmHg per 10 kg weight loss
Eat a diet rich in fruit, vegetables and low-fat dairy products, and low in saturated and total fat	8–14 mmHg
Reduce salt consumption to less than 2.4 g sodium (less than 6 g salt)	2–8 mmHg
Take regular aerobic activity (e.g. brisk walking for at least 30 minutes a day)	4–9 mmHg
Drink 21 units a week or less (men) or 14 units a week or less (women)	2–4 mmHg

Source: Williams and colleagues.

people do much better than this – especially when they combine several changes (Table 7.1). Around half of people who follow a low-calorie diet show a reduction in blood pressure of at least 5/5 mmHg. In around a third of people who reduce their salt consumption from 10 grams a day to five grams a day, blood pressure falls by at least 5/5 mmHg. Nevertheless, most people also need to take blood pressure-lowering drugs (antihypertensives).

Doctors can choose from among a wide range of antihypertensives, including ACE inhibitors, diuretics, beta-blockers and calcium channel blockers. There's not space to discuss the pros and cons of each here. So, talk to your doctor and check out NHS Choices and patient groups' websites. This therapeutic diversity means, for example, if you suffer, or are at risk of, a side effect – such as asthma with beta-blockers, a persistent dry cough with ACE inhibitors, increases in potassium and sugar in your blood with some diuretics, or flushed face or headaches with calcium channel blockers – doctors can usually find an alternative.

Beta-blockers and asthma

Doctors prescribe drugs called beta-blockers for, among other conditions, hypertension, some anxiety symptoms and glaucoma. (In glaucoma, pressure exerted by fluids inside the eye damages the nerves carrying signals from the light-sensitive retina at the back of the eye to the brain. Untreated glaucoma can lead to blindness.) Beta-blockers cause airways to narrow. In healthy people taking beta-blockers, the narrowing isn't enough to cause respiratory symptoms. However, in people with asthma the narrowing may provoke an attack. Enough beta-blocker can even reach the bloodstream from eye drops used to treat glaucoma to trigger an attack.

Antihypertensives when taken regularly, Neal and colleagues found, reduced the risk of stroke by 20–39 per cent, CHD by 19–20 per cent and major cardiovascular events (stroke, MI, heart failure or death from any cardiovascular cause) by 15–28 per cent, depending on the drug and dose. However, a single antihypertensive controls blood pressure adequately in only 20–30 per cent of patients, Gradman remarks. So, most people need at least two antihypertensives that have complementary mechanisms. Many people need at least three. That's one reason why it's so important to change your lifestyle: you may be less likely to need multiple drugs. Lifestyle modification can lower blood pressure as much as a single antihypertensive, Williams and colleagues remark.

Tackling salt

According to the British Dietetic Association (BDA), the average UK adult eats around 8.6 g of salt a day – that's about two teaspoons. The recommended intake for adults is 6 g of salt a day. Eating too much salt increases your risk of hypertension. While everyone needs to control their consumption, it's especially important for heart attack survivors and other people with cardiovascular disease.

You can tell that some snacks are salty. But many foods contain 'hidden salt': your taste buds won't warn you. For instance, some breads and breakfast cereals contain considerable amounts of salt. Indeed, salt already added to food accounts for three-quarters of our intake.

So, check the label and try to stick to low salt foods (Table 7.2). The BDA advises choosing meals and sandwiches with less than 0.5 g of sodium (1.25 g salt) per meal. For individual foods – such as soups and sauces – choose foods with under 0.3 g of sodium (0.75 g) per serving. Use as little salt as you can during cooking, banish the cellar from the table and, the BDA recommends, ask restaurants and take-aways for 'no salt'. You quickly get used to the taste.

Some labels list the sodium, rather than salt, content. Chemically, table salt is sodium chloride. To convert sodium to salt – multiply by 2.5. So, 0.4 g of sodium is 1 g of salt. You can convert salt to sodium by dividing by 2.5.

Table 7.2 Salt levels in food

Level	Salt content	Sodium content
High	More than 1.5 g per 100 g	More than 0.6 g per 100 g
Medium	0.3 g–1.5 g per 100 g	0.1–0.6 g per 100 g
Low	0.3 g or less per 100 g	0.1 g or less per 100 g

Sally's story

Sally, an obese 56-year-old office manager, always seemed to be on a diet, knew she drank more than she should and regularly snacked on peanuts and crisps as she watched every soap on television. During a routine check-up, her nurse diagnosed hypertension. Three months later, her first drug hadn't lowered her blood pressure enough. Then a couple of days after starting on two antihypertensives, she was admitted to hospital suffering unstable angina. It proved a life-changing event. Eight months later, she's lost almost 20 kg in weight, curtailed her drinking and dramatically cut back her salt consumption. Her blood pressure fell by 11/9 mmHg and she's only taking one antihypertensive. Sally hasn't suffered an angina attack since and she wants to work with her GP to come off antihypertensives altogether. 'I just wish I'd made the changes before,' she says.

A healthy diet

Mother was right: you are what you eat. Humans didn't evolve to chomp on foods high in fat and calories and low in fruit and vegetables while being couch potatoes. Trevathan and colleagues note that between 50 and 80 per cent of the diets of hunter–gatherers derives from plants and, as a result, is rich in whole grains and low in saturated fats. Furthermore, hunter–gatherers need to keep moving to search for food and water. So is it any wonder that heart disease, diabetes and obesity are common in industrial societies?

Despite their healthy diets and active lifestyle, injury and disease meant that our ancestors typically lived much shorter lives than their descendents today. Nevertheless, at least 8 per cent of people in typical hunter–gatherer societies survive beyond 60 years of age. Even allowing for the shorter life expectancy, hypertension and heart disease are relatively rare.

There's now no doubt that a healthy diet – reminiscent of our hunter–gatherer ancestors – is good for our heart. For example, Akbaraly and colleagues examined the dietary habits of 7,319 British civil servants, using the Alternative Healthy Eating Index (AHEI). The AHEI scores consumption of nine components of your diet: vegetables; fruit; nuts and soy; white or red meat; trans fat; polyunsaturated or saturated fat; fibre; multivitamin use; and alcohol. The researchers split the civil servants into three groups based on their AHEI score.

During the 18-year long study, the third who ate the most healthy diets were 24 per cent less likely to die from any cause and 42 per cent less likely to die from cardiovascular disease as those in the lowest third. Eating nuts and soy combined with a 'moderate' alcohol intake (half to one-and-a-half US drinks – a US 'drink' is just under two British units – for women; one-and-a-half to two-and-a-half for men) appeared to make the greatest contribution to the decreased death toll.

The NHS suggests making sure you eat at least five portions of vegetables and fruit each day following an MI. For example, increasing fruit and vegetable consumption from two to seven portions daily lowers blood pressure by around 7/3 mmHg in people with hypertension. If the increase in fruit and vegetables is combined with an increase in low-fat dairy products and reduction of total and saturated fat, blood pressure may decline by 11/6 mmHg.

We'll focus on the three 'F's that form the foundation of a heart-healthy diet: fat, fish and fibre. There's only space to skim the surface of a healthy diet. If you want to know more or if you want advice on changing other aspects of your diet, your GP can refer you to a dietician or you can check out the comprehensive advice on the BDA website. And don't be tempted to follow a 'celebrity' or popular diet without checking first.

Fat – cholesterol and beyond

Atherosclerotic plaques are rich in cholesterol. However, the amount of cholesterol in your blood depends more on the amount of saturated fat – animal fat in meat, full-fat dairy products, cakes, biscuits, pastries and so on – you eat than the amount of cholesterol. Indeed, few foods contain high levels of cholesterol: eggs, liver, kidneys and prawns are some notable exceptions. Diet accounts for only around a third of the cholesterol in the body.

So, the idea that you need to eat no more than three eggs a week is now outdated. Eggs are one of the most nutritious foods – which makes sense when you think how well they support growth. It's fine to go to work on an egg, as part of a balanced diet. You only need to cut down on cholesterol-rich food if advised to do so by your GP or a registered dietician.

Rather than worrying about cholesterol, focus on saturated fat. The liver converts saturated fat into cholesterol. Eating foods rich in saturated fat also slows the rate at which your body removes cholesterol. However, the BDA notes that most people in the UK eat about 20 per cent more than the recommended levels: no more than 20 g and 30 g of saturated fat a day for women and men respectively. So, eat less food high in saturated fat. The BDA points out that foods with more than 5 g of saturated fat per 100 g are high in fat. Foods with 1.5 g or less saturated fat per 100 g are low in fat. Table 7.3 suggests some ways you could cut your consumption of saturated fat.

Table 7.3 Foods high in saturated fat and some low-fat alternatives

	Foods to avoid (high in saturated fat)	Low-fat alternative
Snacks	Crisps and savoury snacks cooked in oil	Fresh or dried fruit, a handful of nuts
Fats for cooking and spreading	Lard, dripping, ghee, cream and butter	Olive, sunflower, soya or rapeseed (blended vegetable) oils, margarines and spreads
Meat	Fatty products (sausages, burgers, pâté, salami, meat pies and pasties)	Lean cuts of meat and mince (check labels or ask the butcher) with the fat trimmed off, skinless chicken and turkey, vegetarian options (lentils, chick peas and soya)
Fish	Deep fried (e.g. take-away) fish and chips	Oily fish such as salmon, mackerel, sardines
Sauces	Creamy or cheesy sauces	Tomato- or vegetable-based sauces
Dairy	Full-fat varieties	Skimmed (or at least semi-skimmed) milk; reduced-fat cheddar and low-fat yoghurt; try grating cheese or using a strong-flavoured variety, which may mean you need to use less

Source: British Dietetic Association.

The trans fat danger

Gram for gram, trans fatty acids increase heart disease risk more than saturated fats. Unfortunately, numerous foods – including cheese, cream, beef, lamb and mutton – contain trans fatty acids. Heating vegetable oil to fry foods and food processing also create trans fatty acids. Hydrogenation, for example, turns vegetable oils into solid or semi-solids containing trans fats. Biscuits, pies, cakes and some margarines and other spreads often contain hydrogenated (also called trans-unsaturated) fats. So, look for 'low in trans' or 'virtually trans free' foods and check the ingredients. Foods containing hydrogenated fats or hydrogenated vegetable oils almost always have trans fatty acids. Remember that the higher up the list an ingredient appears, the more of that ingredient the food contains.

Changing to a low-fat diet can be tough. But it's worth making the effort. If these changes don't reduce your blood cholesterol level sufficiently, you may need to take medicines. However, these are an addition to a low fat diet. They're not a replacement.

Fish and omega-3 fatty acids

Life inside the Arctic Circle is tough. Few plants survive. So, the traditional diet of first-nation Arctic people consists almost entirely of fish, seals and other meats. Yet they seem to be less vulnerable to several diseases, including diabetes, heart disease, arthritis and asthma, than people in Western countries.

Eventually, researchers resolved this paradox. These traditional diets are high in fish and animals that eat marine life. Some fish oils (n-3, also called omega-3, fatty acids) appear to reduce inflammation, increase HDL, cut triglycerides and lower blood pressure. So, eating oily fish helps lowers your risk of cardiovascular disease. And there are other benefits. Oily fish, the BDA points out, keep your joints healthy. Omega-3 fatty acids are also important for memory, intellectual performance and some behaviours.

Omega-3 fatty acids – specifically docosahexaenoic acid (DHA) and eicosapentaenoic acid (EPA) – seem to be responsible for much of the benefit produced by oily fish. We can make omega-3 fatty acids from another fat (alpha-linolenic acid) in green leafy vegetables, nuts, seeds and their oils. But it's a slow process. So, it's a good idea to boost levels by eating fish and seafood high in omega-3 fatty acids, such as tuna, salmon, herring, pilchards, mackerel, rainbow trout, dogfish, shrimp and crab. It's better to eat fresh fish. If you're eating canned fish, check the label to make sure processing hasn't depleted the omega-3 oils. It's also worth trying to check that the fish comes from sustainable stocks (<www.fishonline.org>).

The BDA advises that adults and children over 12 years of age should eat two portions of fish per week (a portion is about 140 g after cooking). One of these meals should be an oily fish. The BDA estimates that this will provide the equivalent of about 450 mg EPA or DHA per day. If you've already suffered a heart attack, NICE advises eating at least 7 g of omega-3 fatty acids per week from two to four portions of oily fish.

If at first you don't like the taste, don't give up without trying a few recipes. For an island nation, our tastes in fish are remarkably conservative. But if you really can't stomach the taste of oily fish you could try a supplement. The BDA suggests taking a supplement that provides the recommended amount in two to four portions of fish (450–900 mg EPA or DHA). NICE adds that if you've had a heart attack within the past 3 months and you can't consume sufficient omega-3 fatty acids, you could take at least 1 g daily of omega-3 supplement for up to 4 years.

It's worth buying omega-3 supplements from a reputable company that certifies that its products are free of toxic heavy metals – such as mercury, lead and cadmium – which some fish concentrate. High doses of omega-3 fatty acids may increase the risk of bleeding. So if you bruise easily, have haemophilia or another bleeding disorder or take blood-thinning medications (including aspirin, warfarin and clopidogrel) you should speak to your doctor first. Omega-3 supplements may also increase blood sugar levels. So, again, if you have type 2 diabetes, ask your doctor before taking omega-3 or fish oil supplements.

Fibre and whole grains

Dietary fibre (roughage) is the part of plants that humans can't digest. There are two main types:

- Insoluble fibre remains largely intact as it moves through your digestive system, but eases defecation.

- Soluble fibre dissolves in water in the gut, forming a gel that soaks up fats.

Regularly eating foods rich in soluble fibre – including oats and oat bran, fruit and vegetables, nuts, beans and pulses such as peas, soya, lentils and chickpeas – helps reduce the amount of saturated fat you absorb from your diet. Dieticians recommended that adults should eat at least 18 g of fibre a day. Currently, the average UK adult eats between 12 g and 14 g a day.

Whole grains are an especially good source of fibre. Grains are the seeds of cereals, such as wheat, rye, barley, oats and rice. An outer layer that is rich in fibre (bran) covers the 'germ', which is packed with nutrients. Finally, the central area (endosperm) is rich in starch. Food manufacturers refine grain by removing the bran and germ, and keep the white endosperm. This removes most of nutritional value: whole grain contains up to 75 per cent more nutrients than refined cereals, the BDA points out.

Regularly eating whole grain as part of a low fat diet and a healthy lifestyle cuts the risk of heart disease and type 2 diabetes by up to 30 per cent. Whole grains even help you stay slim by releasing sugar slowly into your blood. This, along with the high fibre content, means that you feel fuller for longer. So, you're less likely to snack during the morning after a breakfast of porridge and whole-grain bread than after one of refined cereals and white toast. Yet 95 per cent of adults in the UK don't eat enough whole grains. Nearly a third don't eat any. The BDA suggests that you should aim to get at least half your starchy carbohydrates from whole grains, which means around two to three servings a day. Try eating more foods with 'whole' in front of the grain's name – such as whole wheat pasta and whole oats.

Drugs that lower lipids

Medicine usually advances in small steps. Occasionally, however, a study is so important that treatment changes almost overnight. In the early 1990s, doctors knew that cholesterol filled atherosclerotic plaques. But there wasn't any firm evidence that cutting blood cholesterol levels saved lives. Then, in 1994, *The Lancet* reported results from the Scandinavian Simvastatin Survival Study (4S).

4S included 4,444 people with serum cholesterol levels between 5.5 and 8.0 mmol/L who either had angina or had previously suffered a heart attack. All those in the study ate a lipid-lowering diet and received simvastatin or placebo. After, on average, almost five and a half years, simvastatin reduced total cholesterol by 25 per cent, cut LDL by 35 per cent and increased HDL levels by 8 per cent. Deaths overall fell by 30 per cent, while the risk of death from heart disease declined by 42 per cent. The number of people who experienced at least one major coronary event – including non-fatal heart attacks – declined by 34 per cent. Simvastatin also reduced revascularization procedures by 37 per cent.

Since 4S, numerous studies confirmed that lipid-lowering drugs – several related medicines followed in the wake of simvastatin, collectively called statins – improve blood lipid levels. Overall, statins lower LDL by 18–55 per cent, raise HDL levels by 4–9 per cent and cut triglyceride levels by 7–30 per cent. According to the Cholesterol Treatment Trialists' Collaboration, over an average of 4.8 years, each 1.0 mmol/litre reduction in LDL cut overall mortality by 10 per cent. Deaths due to CHD and other cardiac causes fell by 20 per cent and 11 per cent, respectively. Lipid lowering drugs are now a mainstay of heart disease prevention before and after an MI. If you've suffered a MI, NICE suggests aiming for a total cholesterol level of under 4.0 mmol/litre or LDL less than 2.0 mmol/L, whichever of the two represents the greater decrease in your lipid levels.

Statins can cause side effects, including headache, dizziness, changes in the enzymes produced by your liver, rash, myalgia (muscle pain and cramps) and rhabdomyolysis, where muscle damage releases a protein called myoglobin (see page 49) into the blood stream. Excessive levels of myoglobin can lead to kidney damage. But these side effects are relatively uncommon. Fewer than one person in every 1,000 taking 40 mg of simvastatin daily develops myopathy (muscle weakness and cramps with CK [page 49] ten times normal), for example. But if you feel unwell while taking statins, see your GP.

Drugs that boost HDL

Statins, the most widely used lipid-lowering drug, are often less effective at increasing HDL than other medicines, called fibrates and niacin. Several lifestyle changes also boost HDL, O'Keefe and colleagues note, including quitting smoking, weight loss and exercise. HDL-friendly diets are high in unsaturated fats, omega-3 fatty acids, and lean protein, with limited amounts of high glycaemic index carbohydrates (e.g. sugar, white bread and certain breakfast cereals). Many food labels now state if the food has a low glycaemic index, and Diabetes UK produced a list (<www.diabetes.org.uk/Guide-to-diabetes/Food_and_recipes/The-Glycaemic-Index>).

So if your main problem is low HDL, your doctor may suggest fibrates or niacin rather than a statin in addition to lifestyle changes. If you have both high LDL and low HDL, your doctor may suggest combining a fibrate or niacin with a statin.

Your good health? Alcohol and heart attacks

The UK is a nation of heavy drinkers. But excessive drinking isn't just a problem for bingeing teenagers or homeless drunks. According to the Office for National Statistics, 41 per cent of men in managerial and professional households drank more than four units on at least one day in the previous week. And in these households, 35 per cent of women drank more than three units on at least one day in the week before interview. This compares to 34 per cent of men and 23 per cent of women in 'routine' work or manual-work households.

A very British alcohol unit

In the UK, a 'unit' contain contains 8 g (or 10 ml) of alcohol. A standard bottle (750 ml) of 12 per cent wine contains nine units – so there are three units in a large (250 ml) glass of wine. A pint of 5 per cent beer or cider also contains three units. So, that's 24 g of alcohol. A US 'drink' contains 14 g of alcohol – just under two British units.

Studies showing that drinking small amounts of alcohol cuts the risk of heart disease regularly capture the headlines. Ronksley and colleagues reviewed 84 studies and found that compared to abstaining, drinking 2.5–14.9 g of alcohol a day reduced the risk of:

- CHD by 25 per cent;
- death from cardiovascular disease by 23 per cent;

- death from CHD by 21 per cent;
- stroke by 20 per cent;
- death from stroke by 14 per cent.

Furthermore, O'Keefe and colleagues point out, light-to-moderate alcohol consumption (13–15 g alcohol for women; up to twice this for men) seems to improve the ability of cells to take up glucose after a meal. That's probably why some studies show that alcohol protects your heart most effectively when consumed before or during a meal. Light-to-moderate alcohol consumption also seems to reduce inflammation, boost levels of 'healthy' HDL-cholesterol and, ironically given ubiquitous beer bellies, counter abdominal obesity. One US drink a day (just under two British units) increases HDL by about 5 per cent. Two to three drinks a day increased HDL by 10 per cent. Ethanol (the alcohol in alcoholic drinks) is responsible for most of the benefits. However, red wine is also rich in chemicals called bioflavonoids that are antioxidant, counter blood clots, block a protein called endothelin-1 (which constricts blood vessels) and improve heart rate.

In addition, the US Framingham Heart Study found that men who consumed between eight and 14 'drinks' per week (about 14 to 24 British units) were 59 per cent less likely to develop heart failure than abstainers. No clear benefit emerged among women. The Cardiovascular Health Study found that consuming between seven and 13 US drinks per week (approximately 12 to 23 units) reduced the risk of heart failure by 34 per cent among adults aged at least 65 years. However, other researchers failed to find any benefit, and drinking can lead to alcohol abuse. So, Djoussé and Gaziano comment, people who do not consume any alcohol probably should not start drinking to lower the risk of heart failure.

This sounds good news if you like a tipple. But the amounts are small: 15 g of alcohol a day is less than a pint of beer. Drinking more than this soon becomes hazardous. Ronksley and colleagues found that drinking between 30 g and 60 g of alcohol a day (7.5 units; about two and a half pints of normal strength beer) increases the risk of suffering and dying from a stroke by 15 per cent and 10 per cent, respectively. Drinking more than 60 g increases the risks by 62 per cent and 44 per cent, respectively.

Sesso and colleagues found that drinking just one to three US drinks *a month* increased by 11 per cent the risk that men would develop hypertension, after allowing for other risk factors, such as body mass, exercise, smoking and so on. One drink (roughly two units) a day increased the risk of developing hypertension by 26 per cent. Drinking more than this increased the risk by 29 per cent. In women, the likelihood of developing hypertension initially fell: the risk was 10 per cent lower with five or six US drinks a week. However, the likelihood of developing hypertension was 53 per cent higher among women drinking more than four or five US drinks (7 to about 9 units) a day.

Alcohol's benefits also seem relatively short-lived. So regularly drinking a small amount of alcohol is better than sinking the same amount in a few hours. Ruidavets and colleagues found that over a week, men aged 50 to 59 years in Belfast and France drank similar amounts of alcohol. However, French men spread their consumption more evenly through the week. Men in Belfast tended to drink most of the alcohol on Saturday night. The authors describe this as 'binge' drinking. But the men are not necessarily drinking until they're incapacitated. The authors defined binge drinking as consuming more than 50 g on at least one day a week – that's more than about six units. Nevertheless, men from Belfast were almost 20 times more likely to binge drink than their French counterparts. Binge drinking almost doubled the risk of heart attack and coronary death.

Heavy drinking obviously isn't good for your health. The NHS advises heart attack survivors against binge drinking – more than three alcoholic drinks in one to two hours. In one study of heart attack survivors, binge drinking doubled the risk of death. Furthermore, alcohol causes around 80 per cent of deaths from liver disease, which is now the fifth most common cause of death in England. Alcohol Concern warns that liver disease could overtake stroke and CHD as a cause of death within 10–20 years. Furthermore, heavy drinking over a long time (usually 5–15 years) can, Djoussé and Gaziano comment, directly damage the heart, which enlarges with thin cardiac muscle (dilated cardiomyopathy). The weakened heart muscle pumps inefficiently, leading to heart failure. If you're worried about your drinking call the national drink helpline on 0800 917 8282.

Exercise

When committed couch potatoes run for the bus, their hearts have to work much harder than usual. This sudden bout of exercise can trigger heart attacks. Even if you regularly take mild exercise – such as walking the dog – working especially hard in the garden could trigger an MI. Dahabreh and Paulus found that short-term bouts of exercise increased the risk of suffering a heart attack 3.5-fold and sudden cardiac death about five fold. Even sexual activity almost trebled heart attack risk.

The fitter you are, the less dangerous short bouts of exercise become. Each work-out over a week reduced the risk of heart attack associated with short-term exercise and sexual activity by 45 per cent and sudden cardiac death by 30 per cent. Furthermore, Cardoso and colleagues found that in people with type 2 diabetes, a high level of fitness roughly doubled the chances of having well-controlled blood pressure overnight, a normal pattern of dips in blood pressure over the day (see page 20) and a less stiff aorta. Even moderately fit people showed a healthier pattern than unfit people, although this was less marked than in the very fit.

So how much exercise do you need to keep your heart healthy? The American Heart Association suggests taking at least 10,000 steps a day. You could use a pedometer to ensure you walk far enough. NICE suggests that you should be physically active until you become slightly breathless for between 20 and 30 minutes a day. But you need to exercise regularly. If you've been training regularly for a year, you'll lose about half your cardiovascular fitness in just three months if you stop.

Exercise after a heart attack

If you survived a heart attack some time ago, or if you suffer from angina or have another health issue, you should discuss the amount of physical activity you need with your doctor. For example, people with hypertension shouldn't try isometric exercise such as heavy weight lifting, which can increase blood pressure. So, if you have severe or poorly controlled hypertension, your doctor may suggest avoiding heavy exercise until drugs and lifestyle changes reduce your blood pressure to safe levels.

Immediately after a heart attack, your cardiologist, nurse or physiotherapist will suggest beginning with gentle activity and gradually increasing the intensity. They'll tailor their advice to each individual person. In general, the BHF suggests taking things easy for the first two or three days after your discharge following a heart attack. You should do about the same amount of moving around and exercise indoors as during your last few days in hospital. But make sure that you get enough rest. The BHF suggests (provided your doctor doesn't tell you otherwise) trying to get up, wash and dress, and performing some light tasks around the home, such as making drinks and light snacks, going up and down stairs a few times a day, and gentle walking. Most heart attack survivors can start doing light housework – such as washing up and dusting – when they feel able. After a few weeks, you can probably use a vacuum cleaner, carry the laundry and do light gardening. But avoid digging and heavy lifting. Again if you're in any doubt or you feel unwell at any time, immediately contact your doctor.

Over the next few weeks, you can gradually increase your physical activity. The BHF suggests aiming to do a little bit more each day. But it isn't a challenge. If you feel you can't beat yesterday's performance, don't push yourself. Many people tire easily after a heart attack. The tiredness usually declines as your strength and confidence return. If you suffer angina or feel breathless you must stop and rest. You should always carry your spray or tablets for angina with you and use them as suggested by your doctor.

The BHF suggest that walking – ideally on flat ground – is a good exercise during the first few weeks after a heart attack. (Again, check with the cardiologist or cardiac rehabilitation nurse what's right for you – everyone's different.) You could perform any deep breathing exercises your cardiac rehabilitation team suggested in the fresh air. However, if it's is very hot or very cold, you shouldn't walk outdoors. Exercising after a large meal, when it is very cold or very hot or at high altitudes can place additional strain on your heart. In such circumstances, the BHF suggests walking on the spot, up and down the hallway, or in your local shopping centre or supermarket for the same time instead.

If after a few weeks you feel fine walking, you could talk to your cardiologist, GP or rehabilitation nurse about whether you can start doing more strenuous activities. Provided the medical team agrees, you can probably return to using a treadmill, jogging or swimming (if you swam regularly before your heart attack). However, the pool should be reasonably warm. The BHF advises against taking up swimming after a heart attack. If you are a competitive athlete, you should speak to your doctor before returning to competition.

The NHS also advises against taking part in 'intensely competitive' situations. Whatever your fitness level, if you experience pain in your chest, arm, jaw or shoulder or you are unusually breathless you should stop exercising and see your doctor.

Lose weight

As the bulging waistlines in any high street soon reveal, obesity is common. However, not all fat is equal. As we've seen, abdominal obesity is more harmful for your health than fat elsewhere in your body. In INTERHEART, abdominal obesity increased the risk of suffering a heart attack by between 12 and 62 per cent. So, your waist size can tell you whether your health is at risk. The risk is especially marked in south Asian people (Table 7.4).

Table 7.4 Waist sizes linked to health risk

	Waist size putting health at risk	Waist size putting health at high risk
Men	Over 94 cm (37 inches)	Over 102 cm (40 inches)
Women	Over 80 cm (32 inches)	Over 88 cm (35 inches)
South Asian men		Over 90 cm (36 inches)
South Asian women		Over 80 cm (32 inches)

Source: British Heart Foundation.

Unfortunately, losing weight is not easy – whatever the latest fad diets would have you believe. After all, millions of years of evolution drive us to consume food in times of feast to help us survive during times of famine. And you can't stop eating as you can quit smoking. However, the following tips may help:

- Set yourself a realistic target. The NHS suggests around 0.5 kg a week following an MI.
- Your exercise programme and heart-healthy diet will help you lose weight after a heart attack. So, try to stick to them.

- Keep a food diary and record everything you eat and drink for a couple of weeks. It's often easy to see where you inadvertently pile on the extra calories: the odd biscuit here, the extra glass of wine or full-fat latte there. It all adds up. A food diary can also help you see if you're eating fatty or high salt food without realising.
- Set specific goals. Don't say that you want to lose weight: rather, resolve to lose, for example, 10 kg (about two stone). You should agree a target with your GP, cardiologist or rehabilitation nurse.

Don't let a slip-up derail your diet. Try to identify why you indulged – what were the triggers? A particular occasion? Or do you comfort eat? Once you know why you slipped you can develop strategies to stop the problem in the future.

If all this fails, try talking to your GP. A growing number of medicines may help kick-start your weight loss. None of these drugs is a magic cure for being overweight. You'll still need to change your lifestyle. However, they help put you on the right course towards weight loss.

Vaccination

Influenza isn't a bad cold. Flu is potentially fatal, especially for older people and those with certain serious medical conditions. For example, the Department of Health estimates that suffering from chronic heart disease increases the chances of someone between the ages of 6 months and 64 years dying from flu almost 11-fold. So it's important to get your flu jab if, for example:

- you have a heart problem, such as chronic heart failure or you need regular treatment for angina or ischaemic heart disease;
- you have a chest complaint or breathing difficulties;
- you have kidney disease;
- you have suffered a stroke or a transient ischaemic attack ('mini-stroke') in the past;
- you have diabetes.

The Department of Health's website (<www.dh.gov.uk/en/Publichealth/Flu/index.htm>) lists who should be vaccinated. Your close family should also consider having the seasonal jab. However, government figures suggest that only around 73 per cent of people aged at least 65 years were immunized with the winter flu vaccine during 2010–2011, and only around half of high-risk people (including those with heart disease) below 65 years of age. If you are in a vulnerable group or caring for a high-risk person, your GP surgery should offer you a flu jab. If you feel you should have the jab but aren't offered it, speak to your GP or practice nurse.

Complementary therapy

Few areas of medicine attract as much controversy as complementary and alternative therapies. They're undoubtedly popular. Greenfield and colleagues found that one in 10 people with CHD attending hospital for their 12-month follow up in the West Midlands used complementary and alternative medicine. Just over a quarter of these used complementary and alternative medicine to manage their cardiac problems. Most used it for other illnesses.

Furthermore, many people find complementary therapies relaxing. We've seen that emotions and stress can trigger angina. So, it's not surprising that people find aromatherapy, Reiki and other massage techniques, and relaxation therapies alleviate angina symptoms and reduce stress – which is another heart attack risk factor. Yoga and exercise both seem to improve mood and reduce anxiety. But yoga may improve mood and reduce anxiety more than the same amount of exercise gained through, for example, walking. (Even so, yoga doesn't replace exercise's cardiovascular benefits.) NICE notes that, overall, relaxation therapies – including progressive muscle relaxation, meditation, yoga, assertiveness training and anger control techniques – reduced systolic blood pressure (by 3.7 mmHg) and diastolic blood pressure (by 3.5 mmHg). A third of people using these techniques show at least a 10 mmHg reduction in systolic blood pressure.

Even the most cynical doctor knows that some herbs can help the heart. In 1785, the English physician William Withering published *An Account of the Foxglove*. A decade before, Withering identified the foxglove as the active plant in a traditional herbal remedy for dropsy – an accumulation of fluid under the skin often caused by heart failure. He derived a drug – digitalis – by slowly drying the leaves of the purple foxglove *(Digitalis purpurea)*, a common British plant, over his study fire. In 1869, chemists purified the active ingredient – called digitoxin – from digitalis. Another species – the white foxglove (*Digitalis lanata*) – yields a related 'cardiac glycoside', digoxin, which works more quickly than digitoxin. Doctors still prescribe digoxin for some cases of heart failure and atrial fibrillation. The autumn crocus (*Colchicum autumnale*) yields colchicine, still used as a gout treatment.

Nevertheless, many doctors and nurses remain cynical about complementary medicine more generally, especially those therapies they regard as scientifically untenable. Certainly few complementary therapies undergo the same rigorous scrutiny as modern medicines. But clinical studies are expensive and pharmaceutical companies fund most trials, so this lack of studies isn't that surprising. It's worth remembering that no evidence of effectiveness isn't necessarily the same as evidence of no effect.

Cynics add that the placebo effect accounts for most of the benefits produced by complementary medicines. In other words, if you think that treatment will work and you relax during the therapy session, you'll probably feel better. However, the placebo effect also contributes to the benefits of conventional medicines. Because of this, many studies compare a conventional drug to a placebo, which looks the same but doesn't contain active ingredients. (We've looked at several examples in this book.) Including a placebo reduces the risk that, for example, people who change their lifestyle because they're taking part in a study or they're having more frequent contact with doctors while they're in the study will bias the results. Ideally, neither the patient nor the doctor knows whether the treatment is active or a placebo (a 'double-blind' study.) So you need to decide whether the evidence for a complementary therapy convinces you, keep taking your conventional treatments and ensure it won't do you any harm.

A common misconception

There's a common misconception that because complementary therapies are natural they are, therefore, safe. But even high doses of vitamins can be dangerous. In 1596, Dutch sailors exploring the Arctic island of Novaya Zembla fell dangerously ill after eating polar bear liver. Three sailors lost their skin 'from head to foot'. Many subsequent expeditions fell victim to the same malady. We now know that polar bear livers contain very high levels of vitamin A. You're unlikely to eat enough vitamin A to suffer the same fate, but it remains a sobering reminder that while sufficient vitamins and minerals are essential for health, excessive levels can be dangerous.

Some supplements may even increase MI risk. The NHS suggests that heart attack survivors should not take supplements of beta-carotene (which the body converts into vitamin A), because they may increase the risk of further cardiovascular events. Bolland and colleagues found that over an average of four years people taking a calcium supplement were 27 per cent more likely to suffer a heart attack. Overall, treating 1,000 people with calcium for five years would cause 14 extra MIs, 10 extra strokes and 13 extra deaths, while preventing 26 fractures. And certain herbs and supplements can interact with other drugs. For example:

- Asian ginseng is unsuitable for diabetics.
- St John's wort (used for depression) can interact with the contraceptive pill and with warfarin.
- Garlic can 'thin the blood' and interfere with some HIV treatments.
- Vitamin E (probably at doses greater than 400 international units a day) can interact with anticoagulant or antiplatelet medications, such as aspirin and warfarin, and increase the risk of bleeding. The risk is especially marked in people with a low intake of vitamin K, which is essential for normal blood clotting.
- Vitamin E combined with other antioxidants – such as vitamin C, selenium and beta-carotene – can attenuate the rise in HDL in people taking simvastatin and niacin.

Not all products include the detailed information you need to take the supplement safely. So talk to your doctor or cardiac nurse before trying a complementary treatment. And speak to a pharmacist if you want to buy a herbal treatment. Rather than treating yourself using herbs, it's advisable to consult a qualified medical herbalist.

Vitamins and dietary supplements

In the early 1990s, a spate of studies suggested that vitamin E might cut the risk of heart disease. In one trial that included around 90,000 nurses, high intakes of vitamin E seemed to reduce the risk of heart disease by 30–40 per cent. And it seemed plausible. Vitamin

E mops up tissue-damaging free radicals, reduces inflammation and inhibits platelet aggregation. Indeed, when I attended a meeting of US cardiologists in the mid-1990s, one speaker asked how many doctors suggested that their patients take vitamin E. A few – probably less than a fifth it seemed to me – raised their hand. He then asked how many doctors and their families took vitamin E. Well over half voted yes.

This enthusiasm now seems premature. The HOPE study, which followed almost 10,000 people at high risk of heart attack or stroke for 4.5 years, found that 400 international units a day of vitamin E did not protect against cardiovascular events or hospitalizations for heart failure or chest pain compared with a placebo. More recently, Sesso and colleagues found that over an average of 8 years, neither vitamin E (400 international units every other day) nor 500 mg vitamin C daily alone or in combination reduced the number of major cardiovascular events, heart attacks, strokes or deaths from cardiovascular causes compared with placebo in 15,000 healthy doctors aged at least 50 years. On the other hand, men taking vitamin E were 74 per cent more likely to suffer a haemorrhagic stroke. Some doctors believe that vitamin E may be more effective in younger people taking higher doses. But further research is needed.

Other supplements, according to some studies at least, may protect against heart disease. We've already seen that omega-3 supplements can offer an option for people who can't stomach oily fish. Wang found that moderate-to-high doses (approximately 1000 international units a day) of vitamin D reduced the risk of cardiovascular disease by 10 per cent. Furthermore, high levels of homocysteine (a chemical involved in several important chemical reactions in the body) increase heart disease risk. Low levels of folic acid (vitamin B_9), pyridoxine (vitamin B_6) and cobalamin (vitamin B_{12}) can increase homocysteine levels in the blood. B vitamin supplements reduce homocysteine levels. But Clarke and colleagues analysed eight studies showing that although B vitamin supplements lowered homocysteine by about 25 per cent for about five years, the risk of cardiovascular events, mortality or cancer did not change. Again, more studies are needed.

As a final example, garlic may lower levels of fat in the blood, reduce the likelihood of blood clots, mop up tissue-damaging free radicals and improve the function of the inner lining of the blood vessels. However, not all studies found that garlic or garlic preparations lower fats sufficiently to reduce cardiovascular risk, Gorinstein and co-authors remark. In part, the differences reflect the use of various preparations, some of which may include other active ingredients or differ in how much reaches the blood. So if you want to use garlic (or any other supplement) buy a reputable brand, ideally check that it's working and try to stick to the same product.

Drawing conclusions is difficult. The evidence and the rigour of the studies are mixed and, as the garlic debate shows, several factors can influence the results. There's no doubt that by far the best way to get vitamins and minerals is to eat a healthy mixed diet. It's probably safe to take a standard multivitamin supplement. (But check with your doctor or pharmacist that it won't interact with your medicines.) On the other hand, avoid high doses of a vitamin unless you're discussed the risks and benefits with your doctor or dietician.

Only limited scientific evidence supports many complementary therapies and conventional health-care professionals are often cynical. But there's no doubt some people feel that they benefit. As we've seen, emotions and stress can trigger angina and heart attacks. So that's not a benefit to lightly dismiss. Whatever treatment you decide, regard the therapy as *complementary* – not alternative. Find a reputable, qualified therapist and consider keeping a diary of your symptoms to see if, for example, you suffer fewer angina attacks. Don't stop taking your conventional medicines, and make sure your nurse, doctor and therapist knows.

8

Heart attacks and the family

The ripples from any serious disease can spread throughout the family. For example, after a heart attack, the partner and other family members may treat the patient with kid gloves. But to recover fully, a person who has had a heart attack needs to get back in the swing of everyday life. Walking the tightrope between not letting you do anything and allowing you to do too much, dealing with the practical problems, as well as the sobering thought you might have died and their fears for the future, often make the days and weeks after your heart attack especially difficult for your family.

Your partner shoulders an especially heavy burden. He or she may fear being left alone if you die, may may worry that sex could trigger an attack and may feel guilty about taking any personal time out. This can, obviously, place a considerable strain on your relationship – just when you need your partner the most.

So you, your partner and, when appropriate, other family members should discuss what you should do, and when, with the cardiac rehabilitation team, GP and the district or cardiac nurses. In some parts of the country, you and your partner may receive a visit from a cardiac liaison or BHF nurse, who can answer your questions and offer advice on how to reduce your risk of further heart disease. Every family is different. But this chapter looks at some suggestions that may help make life easier for your family as well as how your family can help you.

Heart-warming relationships

John Donne famously commented that 'no man is an island' – and friends, families and wider social networks are essential for most people to enjoy good health. Several studies suggest that a strong, supportive marriage and other 'satisfying' social relationships improve cardiovascular health, reduce premature death from heart disease and improve your chances of surviving an MI. King and Reis examined 225 people who underwent CABG. Married people were 2.5 times more likely to be alive 15 years after CABG than single people. Among those who were 'highly satisfied' with their marriage, men were 2.7 times, and women 3.9 times, more likely to be alive. Indeed, the quality of the marriage influences several factors linked to progression of heart disease, such as the increase in the size of the left ventricle, blood pressure, chest pain and the amount of calcium in the plaque.

In some ways, these findings aren't surprising. A close family and strong marriage can give patients an especially powerful 'reason to live'. Obviously, people benefit from social, practical and emotional support when they've just been diagnosed with heart disease or while recovering from a MI. Yet, as King and Reis showed, the benefits of marriage persisted for 15 years, which probably reflects the impact of lifestyle changes.

For example, your family's practical and emotional support is invaluable if you are trying to quit smoking, take more exercise, change your diet and take your medicines as prescribed. Your partner can help you adopt a healthy lifestyle, such as changing the shopping list or exercising together. Your partner can ignore bad moods triggered by nicotine withdrawal, boost your motivation to stick to the plan when you feel like quitting and watch for harmful behaviours, such as offering a gentle reminder if you start eating unhealthy food regularly.

On the other hand, single people, especially those who never married, are more likely to die from chronic heart disease or acute coronary syndrome. Social isolation and unsupportive, conflict-ridden relationships also tend to increase cardiovascular morbidity and mortality. Stress between people increases the body's production of chemical messengers that promote inflammation. As mentioned previously, inflammation damages the delicate lining of blood vessels and contributes to plaque rupture. Kiecolt-Glaser and colleagues found that marital conflict and hostility increased levels of these inflammatory messengers compared to couples with more supportive behaviour. Although not heart disease patients, an experimental minor wound healed 40 per cent more slowly in those with 'hostile' marriages.

As this suggests, partners need to tread the fine line between 'nagging' and support. Franks and colleagues found that the spouses' *support* – helping and reinforcing their partner's efforts to tackle unhealthy behaviours – improved the mental health of people in cardiac rehabilitation after a heart attack or CABG. On the other hand, *control* – trying to persuade a partner to adopt healthy behaviours when he or she is unwilling or unable – reduced the likelihood that the survivor would make the changes and undermined mental health.

Helping with medication compliance

Many diseases that increase the risk of heart attack – such as hypertension, raised blood cholesterol and type 2 diabetes – don't cause symptoms. A heart attack may be the first sign that you have, for example, diabetes or hypertension.

This lack of symptoms means that you may not feel any improvement when you take your medicines. Indeed, the side effects of certain drugs can be unpleasant – so you may even feel worse! That's one reason why some people stop taking potentially life-saving medicines (called non-adherence, non-compliance or non-concordance). If you feel that you're developing side effects, speak to your GP: there's usually an alternative.

In other cases, some people may not take their medicines because they feel the drugs are unnecessary or because they deny that they're ill. Other people don't fully appreciate the risks that they're running by not taking their medication. This book, and a full and frank discussion of the risks and benefits with your GP or nurse, should help you understand why you need to take the medicines that could, quite literally, save your life.

Nevertheless, non-adherence is surprisingly common. Yang and colleagues suggested that just over a third of people are non-adherent to oral drugs for diabetes. García Rodríguez and colleagues remark, that each year, one in every 250 patients suffered a non-fatal heart attack because they stopped aspirin.

Overall, Osterberg and Blaschke suggest, patients need to take at least four of every five doses to benefit. Perreault and colleagues found that those who took, on average, 96 per cent of their antihypertensives were 10 per cent less likely to develop coronary artery disease that those who took, on average, 59 per cent of their doses. Furthermore, those who took at least 80 per cent of their statins after one year were 18 per cent less likely to develop cardiovascular disease than those who took less than 20 per cent.

Often, however, poor adherence is unintentional. People may misunderstand treatment instructions, become confused over their medicines – especially if they suffer from other diseases and need to take several drugs – or simply forget. In these cases, adherence aids (such as a box that allows you to organize your tablets day by day) could help, as could simplifying your treatment. (Ask your doctor to check that you really need all the drugs.) People with physical disabilities may experience difficulties opening packaging or swallowing medication. Pharmacists may be able to suggest alternative packaging or dosing forms, such as avoiding 'child-resistant' pill bottles or using liquid formulations.

Partners, family members and other carers can improve adherence by helping patients establish a routine for taking their medicines. Some partners and family members write a list of the medicines the patient takes and when. The list also means it's easy to remember the medicines if the person suffers another heart attack or needs treatment for another condition. Some medicines can interact with another drug, either causing side effects or undermining the effectiveness of one or both drugs. You could give this list to an unfamiliar doctor (for example if you're on holiday), to A&E staff and to pharmacists if you're buying medication.

Holiday

A few days away helps you and your family relax. But heart attack survivors need to plan their holiday carefully:

- Avoid places that are very hot or very cold. Extremes of temperature can trigger angina and heart attacks.
- Avoid high altitudes. There's less oxygen in the air at high altitudes. So, until you acclimatize (for example, by increasing production of red blood cells) your heart has to work harder.
- Check that the accommodation isn't on too steep a hill or slope, or too far from restaurants, shops and entertainment. (Google Maps with Street View may help.)

- Pollution levels are much higher in some other parts of the world than in the UK: it might be worth checking the air quality of any city you plan to visit.
- Try to avoid stress – after all, a holiday is supposed to be a time to relax. The BHF suggests going to a destination that you've visited recently before to reduce the risk of unwelcome surprises.
- Make sure you leave plenty of time to reach the airport or destination.
- Don't carry heavy bags or rush around. People with angina or some other problems may be able to get transport around the terminal.
- You may be able to fly after two or three weeks – sometimes even sooner – if you've recovered from your heart attack without complications. But if you've suffered complications you'll need expert advice. So always check with the cardiologist, GP or rehabilitation nurse (as well as the airline and travel insurance company) that it is safe to fly.
- If you have a pacemaker, you can bypass security systems in shops and airports that could, in rare cases, affect the device. (So don't stand by the security systems at the door when you're waiting for your partner to finish the shopping.) The pacemaker could also set the alarms off. You should have a pacemaker registration card that you should always carried with you. Showing this card should allow you to bypass the systems.
- Check that your travel insurance offers adequate coverage. You should ensure you have information about local emergency and other health services in your destination – ask your tour operator. In the UK, you can check using NHS Choices.
- Check that you take sufficient medicines – remember a repeat prescription won't be available at the end of a phone call. The BHF suggests having a supply in your hand luggage and in your suitcase, and taking a list of all your drugs and doses. Make sure you check for any restrictions about bringing medicines (bought from a pharmacy or on prescription) into your destination. Some painkillers can pose a particular problem in certain countries, for example. You may want to check with the relevant consulate or embassy before you leave home.

Sex and the heart attack survivor

Most people return to their 'normal' sex life after a heart attack. However, sex can, like any physical activity, increase heart rate and blood pressure, which may cause breathlessness (for all the wrong reasons) and chest pain. If you make an uncomplicated recovery, you can usually start having sex again about four weeks after the heart attack, provided you feel comfortable. If you're in any doubt, swallow your embarrassment and check with your cardiologist, GP or rehabilitation nurse. The BHF also provides DVDs and booklets about heart disease and sex life.

If physical activity tends to trigger angina, the BHF suggests not having sex after a heavy meal, keeping the bedroom warm and avoiding cold sheets. It's also a good idea not to drink too much alcohol, to create a relaxing atmosphere and get into a comfortable position. You may find that it helps if your partner takes a more active role. And remember to keep your GTN spray by the bed.

Many heart attack survivors find that their sex drive declines. For example, stress following a heart attack can cause impotence. So a romantic mood and tackling any psychological issues can help reinvigorate a sex life that stalls after a heart attack. Talking to a sympathetic counsellor may help.

In other cases, some drugs (including some antidepressants, beta-blockers and calcium antagonists) or diseases (e.g. diabetes, atherosclerosis and depression) can affect your sex drive or cause impotence. Indeed, cardiovascular disease and erectile dysfunction share many risk factors, including hypertension, raised cholesterol levels, diabetes and smoking. Speak to your GP if you think a medicine or a poorly controlled ailment could be causing impotence. Switching treatment may resolve the problem.

Furthermore, Gratzke and colleagues note, the more extensive your atherosclerosis, the more likely you are to suffer erectile dysfunction. And two-thirds of people with erectile dysfunction have atherosclerosis in their peripheral circulation. In contrast, just over a third of people without erectile dysfunction show these plaques. Indeed, erectile dysfunction usually emerges before symptoms of coronary artery disease, offering an early warning.

Viagra and heart attacks

In some cases, you may be able to take sildenafil (Viagra), tadalafil (Cialis) or vardenafil (Levitra) – which are all phosphodiesterase-5 (PDE-5) inhibitors – for impotence. NICE suggests that doctors can consider a PDE5 inhibitor in people who had a heart attack more than 6 months previously and who are now stable. But never buy Viagra – or any other drug – over the internet. Many internet sites sell fakes, few check to ensure you're a suitable patient and some products contain impurities.

Obviously, if a doctor suggests you should avoid sexual activity – such in some cases of unstable angina or severe heart failure – you shouldn't take drugs for impotence (erectile dysfunction). Furthermore, PDE-5 inhibitors work by dilating the blood vessels supplying the penis. (Indeed, Pfizer originally developed sildenafil to dilate coronary blood vessels to treat angina.) So, combining PDE-5 inhibitors and nitrates could drop your blood pressure to dangerously low levels and you should never use the two together.

A final word to partners

Learn first aid

Ideally, everyone should know basic first aid. But it's especially important for partners of heart attack survivors. For example, people who have survived a MI are more likely to suffer a cardiac arrest. As mentioned earlier, unless defibrillation or cardiopulmonary resuscitation occurs within three to four minutes, a person in cardiac arrest may suffer permanent damage to their brain or other vital organs. You could contact the St John Ambulance or the British Red Cross, or ask your library for details of courses in your area.

Wendy's story

Arthur, a retired engineer, was making cocoa one night when he let out a 'soft moan' and collapsed to the kitchen floor. Wendy, his wife, called 999 immediately. Fortunately, Wendy, a former nurse, knew cardiopulmonary resuscitation and managed to keep Arthur's heart going until the ambulance arrived. The paramedic restarted Arthur's heart with defibrillation and an injection of adrenaline. Arthur now tells everyone that Wendy saved his life.

Look after yourself

Caring for a heart attack survivor can be physically demanding and emotionally draining, especially during the first few weeks while the patient tries to get his or her life back on track. So, to help look after your partner you need to look after yourself.

The BHF suggests trying to rest while the patient is resting and to get a good night's sleep. You should follow the advice offered by the cardiologist, GP or rehabilitation nurse about the patient's activity. Don't offer to do more than this. Your good intentions could hinder their recovery and place an unnecessary burden on your shoulders. Try to limit the number of visitors you have and how long they stay for. And make sure you have time to yourself.

You may also need to honest with yourself. A heart attack can leave your partner mentally and emotionally devastated. He or she may live overshadowed by the fear of another heart attack, may be afraid of dying, may worry about not being able to take part in the activities that were previously enjoyed. Not surprisingly, heart attack survivors may feel depressed, angry, guilty and bad-tempered, which can place a strain on relationships. Partners of people who suffer a heart attack often also harbour feelings of anger, guilt and resentment. Don't bottle these feelings up: as we've seen, conflict between people and in marriages can undermine the patient's long-term prospects. Talk about your feelings to the patient, friends and family or even a counsellor.

Finally, you could think about joining a local or on-line patient group. Groups run by the British Cardiac Patients Association provide advice, information and support to help anyone who has had a heart condition. The BHF hosts an online community (<http://community.bhf.org.uk>), while Carers Direct is a national information, advice and support service for carers in England (<www.nhs.uk/carersdirect>; 0808 802 0202).

Depression and partners

Depression can mean that the person simply can't motivate himself or herself to seek help. Depressed people can feel they're living at the bottom of a deep well: even if they can see the light, it seems faint and distant, and there is no way to climb out. A partner can encourage a depressed or anxious heart attack survivor to seek help. But remember that any ladder you, a doctor or counsellor offers may seem rickety and unstable. You can help engender the confidence the person needs to climb out. Emotional support shows you care and so boosts your partner's feeling of self-worth, both of which can help improve mental health generally and among people with heart disease in particular.

Doctors, scientists and public health officials have made impressive progress tackling heart disease over the last few years. Fewer people than a generation ago now suffer a heart attack and the chances of surviving are better than ever. Nevertheless, heart attacks still kill around one person every six minutes. And despite the medical progress you can't rely on drugs and surgery to save your life. But we've seen throughout this book that you can take steps to reduce your risk of suffering another heart attack and live as full and rich a life as possible after your MI as you did before. An MI doesn't need to break your – or your family's – heart.

Useful addresses

Action on Smoking and Health (ASH)
First Floor, 144–145 Shoreditch High Street
London E1 6JE
Tel.: 020 7739 5902
Website: www.ash.org.uk

Alcohol Concern
64 Leman Street
London E1 8EU
Tel.: 020 7264 0510
Website: www.alcoholconcern.org.uk

AntiCoagulation Europe
PO Box 405
Bromley
Kent BR2 9WP
Tel.: 020 8289 6875
Website: www.anticoagulationeurope.org

Atrial Fibrillation Association
PO Box 1219
Chew Magna
Bristol BS40 8WB
Tel.: 01789 451837
Website: www.atrialfibrillation.org.uk

Blood Pressure Association
60 Cranmer Terrace
London SW17 0QS
Tel.: 0845 241 0989
Website: www.bpassoc.org.uk

British Association for Counselling and Psychotherapy
15 St John's Business Park
Lutterworth
Leics LE17 4HB
Tel.: 01455 883300
Website: www.bacp.co.uk

British Cardiac Patients Association
15 Abbey Road
Bingham
Nottingham NG13 8EE
Tel.: 01223 846845 (helpline: 9 a.m. to 7 p.m., Monday to Saturday);
01949 837070 (general)
Website: www.bcpa.co.uk

British Dietetic Association
Fifth Floor, Charles House
148/9 Great Charles Street
Queensway
Birmingham B3 3HT
Tel.: 0121 200 8080
Website: www.bda.uk.com/index.html
The professional association and trade union for dietitians.

British Heart Foundation
Greater London House
180 Hampstead Road
London NW1 7AW
Tel.: 0300 330 3311 (helpline)
Website: www.bhf.org.uk
For statistics on heart disease: www.bhf.org.uk/heart-health/statistics.aspx

British Register of Complementary Practitioners *see* **Institute for Complementary and Natural Medicine**

Diabetes UK
Macleod House
10 Parkway
London NW1 7AA
Tel.: 020 7424 1000
Website: www.diabetes.org.uk

Heart UK
7 North Road
Maidenhead
Berkshire SL6 1PE
Tel.: 0845 450 5988
Website: www.heartuk.org.uk

Institute for Complementary and Natural Medicine (and **British Register of Complementary Practitioners**)
Can-Mezzanine
32–36 Loman Street
London SE1 0EH
Tel.: 020 7922 7980
Website: www.i-c-m.org.uk

National Health Service (advice on giving up smoking)
Smokefree helpline: 0800 022 4 332
Website: http://smokefree.nhs.uk

Royal College of Psychiatrists
17 Belgrave Square
London SW1X 8PG
Tel.: 020 7235 2351
Website: www.rcpsych.ac.uk
General mental health information for patients:
www.rcpsych.ac.uk/mentalhealthinfoforall.aspx

St John Ambulance
27 St John's Lane
London EC1M 4BU
Tel.: 08700 10 49 50
Website: www.sja.org.uk
Provides first-aid courses around the country.

Stroke Association
Stroke House
240 City Road
London EC1V 2PR
Tel.: 020 7566 0300
Helpline 0303 303 3100 (9 a.m. to 5 p.m., Monday to Friday)
Website: www.stroke.org.uk

Further reading

Craggs-Hinton, C., *Coping with Gout* (new edition). London, Sheldon Press, 2011.
Elliot-Wright, S., *Coping with Type 2 Diabetes*. London, Sheldon Press, 2010.
Greener, M., *Coping With Asthma in Adults*. London, Sheldon Press, 2011.
Smith, T., *Living with Angina*. London, Sheldon Press, 2009.
Smith, T., *Living with Type 1 Diabetes*. London, Sheldon Press, 2010.

References

Introduction

Allam, A. H., Thompson, R. C., Wann, L. S. et al., 'Atherosclerosis in ancient Egyptian mummies: the Horus study', *JACC Cardiovascular Imaging*, 2011, vol. 4, pp. 315–27.

Gutterman, D. D., 'Silent myocardial ischemia', *Circulation Journal*, 2009, vol. 73, pp. 785–97.

Haffner, S. M., Lehto, S., Rönnemaa, T. et al., 'Mortality from coronary heart disease in subjects with type 2 diabetes and in nondiabetic subjects with and without prior myocardial infarction', *New England Journal of Medicine*, 1998, vol. 339, pp. 229–34.

Rosengren, A., Hawken, S., Ounpuu, S. et al.; INTERHEART investigators, 'Association of psychosocial risk factors with risk of acute myocardial infarction in 11119 cases and 13648 controls from 52 countries (the INTERHEART study): case-control study', *The Lancet*, 2004, vol. 364, pp. 953–62.

Yusuf, S., Hawken, S., Ounpuu, S. et al., 'Effect of potentially modifiable risk factors associated with myocardial infarction in 52 countries (the INTERHEART study): case-control study', *The Lancet*, 2004, vol. 364, pp. 937–52.

Chapter 1

Mulder, B. J. M. and van der Wall, E. E., 'Size and function of the atria', *International Journal of Cardiovascular Imaging*, 2008, vol. 24. pp. 713–16.

Chapter 2

Anker, S. D., Voors A., Okonko D. et al., 'Prevalence, incidence, and prognostic value of anaemia in patients after an acute myocardial infarction: data from the OPTIMAAL trial', *European Heart Journal*, 2009, vol. 30, pp. 1331–9.

Cohen, M. C., Rohtla, K. M., Lavery, C. E. et al., 'Meta-analysis of the morning excess of acute myocardial infarction and sudden cardiac death', *American Journal of Cardiology*, 1997, vol. 79, pp. 1512–16.

Corrales-Medina, V. F., Madjid, M. and Musher, D. M., 'Role of acute infection in triggering acute coronary syndromes', *Lancet Infectious Diseases*, 2010, vol. 10, pp. 83–92.

Gutterman, D. D., 'Silent myocardial ischemia', *Circulation Journal*, 2009, vol. 73, pp. 785–97.

Hjalmarson, A., Gilpin, E. A., Nicod, P. et al., 'Differing circadian patterns of symptom onset in subgroups of patients with acute myocardial infarction', *Circulation Journal*, 1989, vol. 80, pp. 267–75.

Nawrot, T. S., Perez, L., Künzli, N. et al., 'Public health importance of triggers of myocardial infarction: a comparative risk assessment', *The Lancet*, 2011, vol. 377, pp. 732–40.

Patel, P. V., Wong, J. L. and Arora, R., 'The morning blood pressure surge: therapeutic implications', *Journal of Clinical Hypertension*, 2008, vol. 10, pp. 140–5.

Rogowski, W., Burch, J., Palmer, S. et al., 'The effect of different treatment durations of clopidogrel in patients with non-ST-segment elevation acute coronary syndromes: a systematic review and value of information analysis', *Health Technology Assessment*, 2009, vol. 13, pp. iii–iv, ix–xi, 1–77.

Tofler, G. H., Muller, J. E., Stone P. H. et al., 'Modifiers of timing and possible triggers of acute myocardial infarction in the Thrombolysis in Myocardial Infarction Phase II (TIMI II) Study Group', *Journal of the American College of Cardiology*, 1992, vol. 20, pp. 1049–55.

Chapter 3

Ahlehoff, O., Gislason, G. H., Lindhardsen, J. et al., 'Prognosis following first-time myocardial infarction in patients with psoriasis: a Danish nationwide cohort study', *Journal of Internal Medicine*, 2011, vol. 270, pp. 237–44.

Arsenault, B. J., Lemieux, I., Després, J. P. et al., 'The hypertriglyceridemic-waist phenotype and the risk of coronary artery disease: results from the EPIC–Norfolk Prospective Population Study', *CMAJ*, 2010, vol. 182, pp. 1427–32.

Cholesterol Treatment Trialists' Collaboration, 'Efficacy and safety of more intensive lowering of LDL cholesterol: a meta-analysis of data from 170 000 participants in 26 randomised trials', *The Lancet*, 2010, vol. 376, pp. 1670–81.

Christoffersen, M., Frikke-Schmidt, R., Schnohr, P. et al., 'Xanthelasmata, arcus corneae, and ischaemic vascular disease and death in general population: prospective cohort study', *BMJ*, 2011, vol. 343, p. d5497.

Coutinho, T., Goel, K., Corrêa de Sá, D. et al., 'Central obesity and survival in subjects with coronary artery disease: a systematic review of the literature and collaborative analysis with individual subject data', *Journal of the American College of Cardiology*, 2011, vol. 57, pp. 1877–86.

Debella, Y. T., Giduma, H. D., Light R. P. and Agarwal, R., 'Chronic kidney disease as a coronary disease equivalent – a comparison with diabetes over a decade', *Clinical Journal of the American Society of Nephrology*, 2011, vol. 6, pp. 1385–92.

Donahoe, S. M., Stewart, G. C., McCabe, C. H. et al., 'Diabetes and mortality following acute coronary syndromes', *JAMA*, 2007, vol. 298, pp. 765–75.

Grundtvig, M., Hagen, T. P., Amrud, E. S. and Reikvam, Å., 'Mortality after myocardial infarction: impact of gender and smoking status', *European Journal of Epidemiology*, 2011, vol. 26, pp. 385–93.

Grundtvig, M., Hagen, T. P., German, M. and Reikvam, Å., 'Sex-based differences in premature first myocardial infarction caused by smoking: twice as many years lost by women as by men', *European Journal of Cardiovascular Prevention and Rehabilitation*, 2009, vol. 16, pp. 174–9.

Haffner, S. M., Lehto, S., Rönnemaa, T. et al., 'Mortality from coronary heart disease in subjects with type 2 diabetes and in nondiabetic subjects with and without prior myocardial infarction', *New England Journal of Medicine*, 1998, vol. 339, pp. 229–34.

Holmqvist, M. E., Wedrén, S., Jacobsson, L. T. et al., 'Rapid increase in myocardial infarction risk following diagnosis of rheumatoid arthritis amongst patients diagnosed between 1995 and 2006', *Journal of Internal Medicine*, 2010, vol. 268, pp. 578–85.

Kannel, W. B., Kannel, C., Paffenbarger, R. S. Jr. et al., 'Heart rate and cardiovascular mortality: the Framingham Study', *American Heart Journal*, 1987, vol. 113, pp. 1489–94.

Kolovou, G. D., Mikhailidis, D. P., Kovar, J. et al., 'Assessment and clinical relevance of non-fasting and postprandial triglycerides: an expert panel statement', *Current Vascular Pharmacology*, 2011, vol. 9, pp. 258–70.

Lemieux, I., Pascot, A., Couillard, C. et al., 'Hypertriglyceridemic waist: a marker of the atherogenic metabolic triad (hyperinsulinemia; hyperapolipoprotein B; small, dense LDL) in men?', *Circulation Journal*, 2000, vol. 102, pp. 179–84.

Logue, J., Murray, H. M., Welsh, P. et al., 'Obesity is associated with fatal coronary heart disease independently of traditional risk factors and deprivation', *Heart*, 2011, vol. 97, pp. 564–68.

Lotufo, P. A., Chae, C. U., Ajani, U. A. et al., 'Male pattern baldness and coronary heart disease: the Physicians' Health Study', *Archives of Internal Medicine*, 2000, vol. 160, pp. 165–71.

Meisinger, C., Döring, A. and Löwel, H., 'Chronic kidney disease and risk of incident myocardial infarction and all-cause and cardiovascular disease mortality in middle-aged men and women from the general population', *European Heart Journal*, 2006, vol. 27, pp. 1245–50.

Mente, A., Yusuf, S., Islam, S. et al., 'Metabolic syndrome and risk of acute myocardial infarction a case-control study of 26,903 subjects from 52 countries', *Journal of the American College of Cardiology*, 2010, vol. 55, pp. 2390–8.

Meune, C., Touzé, E., Trinquart, L. and Allanore, Y., 'High risk of clinical cardiovascular events in rheumatoid arthritis: levels of associations of myocardial infarction and stroke through a systematic review and meta-analysis', *Archives of Cardiovascular Disease*, 2010, vol. 103, pp. 253–61.

Öberg, M., Jaakkola, M. S., Woodward, A. et al., 'Worldwide burden of disease from exposure to second-hand smoke: a retrospective analysis of data from 192 countries', *The Lancet*, 2011, vol. 377, pp. 139–46.

Onusko, E., 'Diagnosing secondary hypertension', *American Family Physician*, 2003, vol. 67, pp. 67–74.

Peters, A. L., 'Patient and treatment perspectives: revisiting the link between type 2 diabetes, weight gain, and cardiovascular risk', *Cleveland Clinic Journal of Medicine*, 2009, vol. 76 (supplement 5), pp. S20–7.

Pound, P., Bury, M. and Ebrahim, S., 'From apoplexy to stroke', *Age and Ageing*, 1997, vol. 26, pp. 331–7.

Roddy, E., 'Revisiting the pathogenesis of podagra: why does gout target the foot?', *Journal of Foot and Ankle Research*, 2011, vol. 4, p. 13.

Rosengren, A., Hawken, S., Ounpuu, S. et al.; INTERHEART investigators, 'Association of psychosocial risk factors with risk of acute myocardial infarction in 11119 cases and 13648 controls from 52 countries (the INTERHEART study): case-control study', *The Lancet*, 2004, vol. 364, pp. 953–62.

Soriano, L. C., Rothenbacher, D., Choi, H. K. and García Rodríguez, L. A., 'Contemporary epidemiology of gout in the UK general population', *Arthritis Research and Therapy*, 2011, vol. 13, p. R39.

Viera, A. J. and Hinderliter, A. L., 'Evaluation and management of the patient with difficult-to-control or resistant hypertension', *American Family Physician*, 2009, vol. 79, pp. 863–9.

Walldius, G. and Jungner, I., 'Apolipoprotein B and apolipoprotein A-I: risk indicators of coronary heart disease and targets for lipid-modifying therapy', *Journal of Internal Medicine*, 2004, vol. 255, pp. 188–205.

Yamazaki, T., Miyazaki, M., Kanase, H. et al., 'Transient hypertension in male adolescents when measured by a woman', *Heart*, 1998, vol. 79, pp. 104–5.

Yusuf, S., Hawken, S., Ounpuu, S. et al., 'Effect of potentially modifiable risk factors associated with myocardial infarction in 52 countries (the INTERHEART study): case-control study', *The Lancet*, 2004, vol. 364, pp. 937–52.

Chapter 4

Alpert, J. S., Thygesen, K., Antman, E. and Bassand, J. P., 'Myocardial infarction redefined – a consensus document of the joint European Society of Cardiology/American College of Cardiology Committee for the Redefinition of Myocardial Infarction', *European Heart Journal*, 2000, vol. 21, 1502–13.

Bassand, J. P., Hamm, C. W., Ardissino, D. et al., 'Guidelines for the diagnosis and treatment of non-ST-segment elevation acute coronary syndromes', *European Heart Journal*, 2007, vol. 28, pp. 1598–660.

Donahoe, S. M., Stewart, G. C., McCabe, C. H. et al., 'Diabetes and mortality following acute coronary syndromes', *JAMA*, 2007, vol. 298, pp. 765–75.

Gutterman, D., 'Silent myocardial ischemia', *Circulation Journal*, 2009, vol. 73, pp. 785–97.

Rogowski, W., Burch, J., Palmer, S. et al., 'The effect of different treatment durations of clopidogrel in patients with non-ST-segment elevation acute coronary syndromes: a systematic review and value of information analysis', *Health Technology Assessment*, 2009, vol. 13, pp. iii–iv, ix–xi, 1–77.

Chapter 5

Dangas, G. and Kuepper, F., 'Restenosis: repeat narrowing of a coronary artery: prevention and treatment', *Circulation Journal*, 2002, vol. 105, pp. 2586–7.

García Rodríguez, L. A., Cea-Soriano, L., Martín-Merino, E. and Johansson, S., 'Discontinuation of low dose aspirin and risk of myocardial infarction: case-control study in UK primary care', *BMJ*, 2011, vol. 343, p. d4094.

Howard, P. A. and Ellerbeck, E. F., 'Optimizing beta-blocker use after myocardial infarction', *American Family Physician*, 2000, vol. 62, pp. 1853–60, 1865–6.

Jacobs, I., Finn, J. C., George, A. et al., 'Effect of adrenaline on survival in out-of-hospital cardiac arrest: a randomized double-blind placebo-controlled trial', *Resuscitation*, 2011, vol. 82, pp. 1138–43.

Magee, K., Sevcik, W. W., Moher, D. and Rowe, B. H., 'Low molecular weight heparins versus unfractionated heparin for acute coronary syndromes, *Cochrane Database of Systematic Reviews*, 2003, issue 1, article CD002132.

Michaels, A. D. and Chatterjee, K., 'Angioplasty versus bypass surgery for coronary artery disease', *Circulation Journal*, 2002, vol. 106, pp. e187–90.

Miner, J. and Hoffhines, A., 'The discovery of aspirin's antithrombotic effects', *Texas Heart Institute Journal*, 2007, vol. 34, pp. 179–86.

O'Donovan, K., 'Prescribing glycoprotein IIb/IIIa inhibitors in ACS', *Nurse Prescribing*, 2011, vol. 9, pp. 391–9.

Perez, M. I., Musini, V. M. and Wright, J. M., 'Effect of early treatment with anti-hypertensive drugs on short and long-term mortality in patients with an acute cardiovascular event', *Cochrane Database of Systematic Reviews*, 2009, issue 4, article CD006743.

Sikri, N. and Bardia, A., 'A history of streptokinase use in acute myocardial infarction', *Texas Heart Institute Journal*, 2007, vol. 34, pp. 318–27.

Unal, B., Critchley, J. A. and Capewell, S., 'Explaining the decline in coronary heart disease mortality in England and Wales between 1981 and 2000', *Circulation Journal*, 2004, vol. 109, pp. 1101–7.

Vlaar, P. J., Svilaas, T., Damman, K. et al., 'Impact of pretreatment with clopidogrel on initial patency and outcome in patients treated with primary percutaneous coronary intervention for ST-segment elevation myocardial infarction: a systematic review', *Circulation Journal*, 2008, vol. 118, pp. 1828–36.

Wang, T. J., Larson, M. G., Levy, D. et al., 'Temporal relations of atrial fibrillation and congestive heart failure and their joint influence on mortality: the Framingham Heart Study', *Circulation Journal*, 2003, vol. 107, pp. 2920–5.

Chapter 6

Benjamin, E. J., Che, P. S., Bild, D. E. et al., 'Prevention of atrial fibrillation: report from a National Heart, Lung, and Blood Institute workshop', *Circulation Journal*, 2009, vol. 119, pp. 606–18.

Boehm, J. K., Peterson, C., Kivimaki, M. and Kubzansky, L. D., 'Heart health when life is satisfying: evidence from the Whitehall II cohort study', *European Heart Journal*, 2011, vol. 32, pp. 2672–7.

Crenshaw, B. S., Ward, S. R., Granger, C. B. et al., 'Atrial fibrillation in the setting of acute myocardial infarction: the GUSTO-I experience. Global Utilization of Streptokinase and TPA for Occluded Coronary Arteries', *Journal of the American College of Cardiology*, 1997, vol. 30, pp. 406–13.

Denollet, J., Schiffer, A. A. and Spek, V., 'General propensity to psychological distress affects cardiovascular outcomes: evidence from research on the type D (distressed) personality profile', *Circulation: Cardiovascular Quality and Outcomes*, 2010, vol. 3, pp. 546–57.

Frasure-Smith, N., Lespérance, F. and Talajic, M., 'Depression following myocardial infarction Impact on 6-month survival', *JAMA*, 1993, vol. 270, pp. 1819–25.

Haffner, S. M., Lehto, S., Rönnemaa, T. et al., 'Mortality from coronary heart disease in subjects with type 2 diabetes and in nondiabetic subjects with and without prior myocardial infarction', *New England Journal of Medicine*, 1998, vol. 339, pp. 229–34.

Jabre, P., Jouven, X., Adner, F. et al., 'Atrial fibrillation and death after myocardial infarction: a community study', *Circulation Journal*, 2011, vol. 123, pp. 2094–100.

Lespérance, F., Frasure-Smith, N., Juneau, M. et al., 'Depression and one-year prognosis in unstable angina', *Archives of Internal Medicine*, 2000, vol. 160, pp. 1354–60.

Pedersen, S. S., Kupper, N. and van Domburg, R. T., 'Heart and mind: are we closer to disentangling the relationship between emotions and poor prognosis in heart disease?', *European Heart Journal*, 2011, vol. 32, pp. 2341–3.

Stewart, S., Hart, C. L., Hole, D. J. et al., 'A population-based study of the long-term risks associated with atrial fibrillation: 20-year follow-up of the Renfrew/Paisley study', *American Journal of Medicine*, 2002, vol. 113, pp. 359–64.

Chapter 7

Akbaraly, T. N., Ferrie, J. E., Berr, C. et al., 'Alternative Healthy Eating Index and mortality over 18 y of follow-up: results from the Whitehall II cohort', *American Journal of Clinical Nutrition*, 2011, vol. 94, pp. 247–53.

Bolland, M. J., Avenell, A., Baron, J. A. et al., 'Effect of calcium supplements on risk of myocardial infarction and cardiovascular events: meta-analysis', *BMJ*, 2010, vol. 341, p. c3691.

Cardoso, C. R. L., Maia, M. D. L., de Oliveira, F. P. et al., 'High fitness is associated with a better cardiovascular risk profile in patients with type 2 diabetes mellitus', *Hypertension Research*, 2011, vol. 34, pp. 856–61.

Cholesterol Treatment Trialists' Collaboration, 'Efficacy and safety of more intensive lowering of LDL cholesterol: a meta-analysis of data from 170,000 participants in 26 randomised trials', *The Lancet*, 2010, vol. 376, pp. 1670–81.

Clarke, R., Halsey, J., Bennett, D. and Lewington, S., 'Homocysteine and vascular disease: review of published results of the homocysteine-lowering trials', *Journal of Inherited and Metabolic Disease*, 2011, vol. 34, pp. 83–91.

Dahabreh, I. J. and Paulus, J. K., 'Association of episodic physical and sexual activity with triggering of acute cardiac events: systematic review and meta-analysis', *JAMA*, 2011, vol. 305, pp. 1225–33.

Djoussé, L. and Gaziano, J. M., 'Alcohol consumption and heart failure: a systematic review', *Current Atherosclerosis Reports*, 2008, vol. 10, pp. 117–20.

Gorinstein, S., Jastrzebski, Z., Namiesnik, J. et al., 'The atherosclerotic heart disease and protecting properties of garlic: contemporary data', *Molecular Nutrition and Food Research*, 2007, vol. 51, pp. 1365–81.

Gradman, A. H., 'Rationale for triple-combination therapy for management of high blood pressure', *Journal of Clinical Hypertension*, 2010, vol. 12, pp. 869–78.

Greenfield, S., Pattison, H. and Jolly, K., 'Use of complementary and alternative medicine and self-tests by coronary heart disease patients', *BMC Complementary and Alternative Medicine*, 2008, vol. 8, p. 47.

Huxley, R. R. and Woodward, M., 'Cigarette smoking as a risk factor for coronary heart disease in women compared with men: a systematic review and meta-analysis of prospective cohort studies', *The Lancet*, 2011, vol. 378, pp. 1297–305.

Law, M., Wald, N., and Morris, J., 'Lowering blood pressure to prevent myocardial infarction and stroke: a new preventive strategy', *Health Technol Assess.*, 2003, 7(31): 1–64.

Neal, B., MacMahon, S., Chapman, N. et al., 'Effects of ACE inhibitors, calcium antagonists, and other blood-pressure lowering drugs: results of prospectively designed overviews of randomised trials', *The Lancet*, 2000, vol. 356, pp. 1955–64.

O'Keefe, J. H., Bybee, K. A. and Lavie, C. J., 'Alcohol and cardiovascular health: the razor-sharp double-edged sword', *Journal of the American College of Cardiology*, 2007, vol. 50, pp. 1009–14.

O'Keefe, J. H., Carter, M. D. and Lavie, C. J., 'Primary and secondary prevention of cardiovascular diseases: a practical evidence-based approach', *Mayo Clinic Proceedings*, 2009, vol. 84, pp. 741–57.

'Randomised trial of cholesterol lowering in 4444 patients with coronary heart disease: the Scandinavian Simvastatin Survival Study (4S)', *The Lancet*, 1994, vol. 344, pp. 1383–9.

Ronksley, P. E., Brien, S. E., Turner, B. J. et al., 'Association of alcohol consumption with selected cardiovascular disease outcomes: a systematic review and meta-analysis', *BMJ*, 2011, vol. 342, p. d671.

Ruidavets, J. B., Ducimetière, P., Evans, A. et al., 'Patterns of alcohol consumption and ischaemic heart disease in culturally divergent countries: the Prospective Epidemiological Study of Myocardial Infarction (PRIME)', *BMJ*, 2010, vol. 341, p. c6077.

Sesso, H. D., Cook, N. R., Buring, J. E. et al., 'Alcohol consumption and the risk of hypertension in women and men', *Hypertension*, 2008, vol. 51, pp. 1080–7.

Sesso, H. D., Buring, J. E., Christen, W. G. et al., 'Vitamins E and C in the prevention of cardiovascular disease in men: the Physicians' Health Study II randomized controlled trial', *JAMA*, 2008, vol. 300, pp. 2123–33.

Trevathan, W. R., Smith, E. O. and McKenna, J. J., *Evolutionary Medicine and Health: New Perspectives*, Oxford University Press, New York, 2008.

Wang, L., Manson, J. E., Song, Y., Sesso, H. D., 'Systematic review: vitamin D and calcium supplementation in prevention of cardiovascular events', *Annals of Internal Medicine*, 2010, vol. 152, pp. 315–23.

Williams, B., Poulter, N. R., Brown, M. J. et al., 'Guidelines for management of hypertension: report of the fourth working party of the British Hypertension Society, 2004-BHS IV', *Journal of Human Hypertension*, 2004, vol. 18, pp. 139–85.

Yusuf, S., Hawken, S., Ounpuu, S. et al., 'Effect of potentially modifiable risk factors associated with myocardial infarction in 52 countries (the INTERHEART study): case-control study', *The Lancet*, 2004, vol. 364, pp. 937–52.

Chapter 8

Franks, M. M., Rook, K. S., Keteyian, S. J. et al., 'Spouses' provision of health-related support and control to patients participating in cardiac rehabilitation', *Journal of Family Psychology*, 2006, vol. 20, pp. 311–18.

García Rodríguez, L. A., Cea-Soriano, L., Martín-Merino, E. and Johansson, S., 'Discontinuation of low dose aspirin and risk of myocardial infarction: case-control study in UK primary care', *BMJ*, 2011, vol. 343, p. d4094.

Gratzke, C., Angulo, J., Chitaley, K. et al., 'Anatomy, physiology, and pathophysiology of erectile dysfunction', *Journal of Sexual Medicine*, 2010, vol. 7, pp. 445–75.

Kiecolt-Glaser, J. K., Loving, T. J., Stowell, J. R. et al., 'Hostile marital inter-actions, proinflammatory cytokine production, and wound healing', *Archives of General Psychiatry*, 2005, vol. 62, pp. 1377–84.

King, K. B. and Reis, H. T., 'Marriage and long-term survival after coronary artery bypass grafting', *Health Psychology*, 2012, vol. 31, 55–62.

Osterberg, L. and Blaschke, T., 'Adherence to medication', *New England Journal of Medicine*, 2005, vol. 353, pp. 487–97.

Perreault, S., Dragomir, A., Roy, L. et al., 'Adherence level of antihyper-tensive agents in coronary artery disease', *British Journal of Clinical Pharmacology*, 2010, vol. 69, pp. 74–84.

Yang, Y., Thumula, V., Pace, P. F. et al., 'Predictors of medication nonad-herence among patients with diabetes in Medicare Part D programs: a retrospective cohort study', *Clinical Therapeutics*, 2009, vol. 31, pp. 2178–88.

Index